RENAL DIET COOKBOOK 2019

The Optimal Nutritious, Low Sodium, Low Salt Recipes with 14 Days Meal Plan to Manage Kidney Disease and Say Goodbye to Dialysis

Dr. Michael Hopkins

Copyright© 2019 By Dr. Michael Hopkins
All Right Reserved.

In no way it is legal to reproduce, duplicate, or transmit any part of this document by either electronic means or printed format. Any recording of this publication is strictly prohibited, and any storage of this material is not allowed unless with a written permission from the publisher. All rights reserved.

The information provided herein is stated to be truthful and consistent, in that any liability, regarding inattention or otherwise, by any usage or abuse of any policies, processes, or directions contained within is the solitary and complete responsibility of the recipient reader. Under no circumstances will any legal liability or blame be held against the publisher for any reparation, damages, or monetary loss due 10 the information herein, either directly or indirectly.

Legal Notice:

This book is copyright protected. This is only for personal use. You cannot amend, distribute, sell, use, quote or paraphrase any part or the content within this book without the consent of the author or copyright owner. Legal action will be pursued if it is breached

Disclaimer notice:

Please 001e the information contained within this document is for educational and enchainment purposes only. Every attempt has been made 10 provide accurate, up to date, complete and reliable information. No warranties of any kind are expressed or implied. Readers acknowledge that the author is not engaging in the rendering of legal, financial, medical or professional advice.

By reading this document, the reader agrees that under no circumstances are we responsible for any losses, direct or indirect, which are incurred as a result of the use of information contained in this document, including but not limited to errors, omissions, or any inaccuracies.

Table of Content

Introduction 2

Chapter 1: Understanding the Renal Diet 4

Concept and etymology 4

Advantages of the renal diet 6

Controlling Your Potassium 9

Controlling Your Phosphorus 10

Controlling your Protein 14

Controlling Your Sodium 15

Controlling Your Fluid Intake 16

What to Eat and what not to eat on a renal diet 18

    What to Eat on a Renal Diet 18

    What Not to Eat on a Renal Diet 22

The Disadvantages of Fast Food for the Renal Patient 24

Meal Plan Tips 25

Renal Diet Main FAQ 27

Chapter 2: Breakfast Recipes 30

Eggs in hole 30

Kidney-friendly French toast 31

Fruit and rolled oat Pancakes 32

Deviled eggs 33

Omelet with onion and apple 34

Breakfast Pork casserole 35

Pepper Quiche 36

Egg Benedict 37

Waffles with cocoa powder 39

Cauliflower and broccoli gratin 40

Wheat Berry bowl 41

Unsalted, Breakfast tortillas 42

Breakfast Couscous 43

Breakfast Custard 44

Breakfast Berry bowl 45

Chapter 3 Lunch Recipes 47

Pork chops with apple 47

Lamb with fruit sauce 48

Slow Cooked chuck roast with onion 49

Pork Tenderloin with cumin 50

Slow cooked chicken with lemon and oregano 51

Oven Baked Halibut 52

Garlic Shrimp 53

Spicy fish with peppers 54

Spicy Chicken Marsala 55

Chicken Curry 56

Steak with onion 57

Shrimp scampi 58

Chicken Paella 59

Beef Kabobs with pepper 60

Chapter 4 Appetizer, snack or salad 62

Egg Rolls 62

Spicy beef meatballs 63

Oven baked Buffalo wings 64

Apple Dip 65

Frozen Cranberry salad 66

Beef Meatloaf 67

Chicken and grape salad 68

Artichoke dip 69

Oven baked okra 70

Stuffed Celery 71

Almond cranberry stuffed celery sticks 72

Cucumber and Onion dip 73

Oven Baked Wontons 74

Oven Baked Eggplant Fries 75

Chapter 5 Dinner Recipes ... 77

Mushroom Pizza ... 77

Chicken Burgers with Sage and Apple ... 78

Turkey Spicy Fajitas ... 79

Pork Souvlaki ... 80

Steamed Talipa Dish with Lemon Juice ... 81

Salmon with Horseradish ... 82

Renal Diet Pilaf ... 83

Lamb Runza ... 84

Onion Pie ... 85

Pepper Pizza ... 86

Baked Dilly Pickerel ... 87

Rice Salad ... 88

Baked Eggplant Tray ... 89

Cranberry Chutney ... 90

Chapter 6 Dessert Recipes ... 92

Apple Cookies ... 92

Raspberry Muffins ... 93

Kidney-friendly Unsalted Pretzels ... 94

Vanilla Custard ... 95

Almond Cookies ... 96

Chocolate Chip Cookies 97

Fruit Compote 98

Puffed Cereal Bars 99

Strawberry Ice-cream 100

Peach Cobbler 101

Zucchini Cake 102

Apple Cake 103

Vanilla Low Potassium Cocoa Cake 104

Blueberry Cones 105

Chapter 7 The 14 Day Meal Plan 106

Conclusion 108

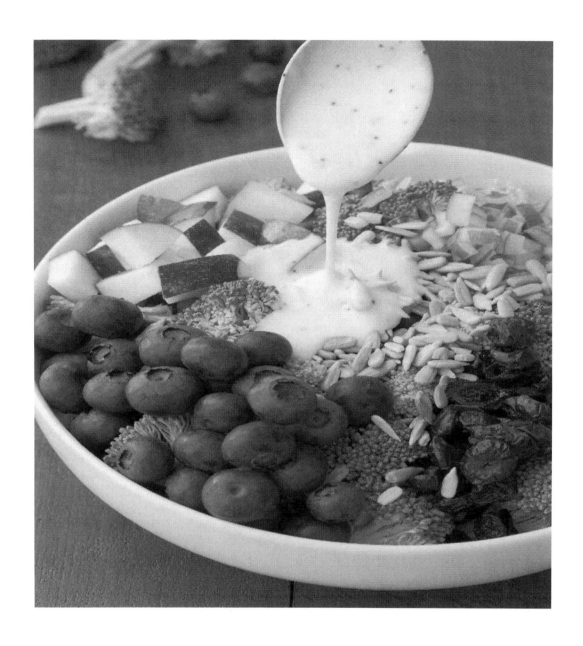

Introduction

Taking the step of adopting a new diet and finding yourself forced to change your lifestyle all of a sudden after being diagnosed with a kidney disease is not a simple step to take. Yet, by deciding the best choices for your health and your body, you can make a huge difference and you will be surprised by the improvement you will notice with a considerable decrease in the painful symptoms you might be experiencing. And this is exactly how this book came to life. So let me first tell you a little bit about the main reason that urged me and encouraged me to write this book.

My story with the renal diet started when a close friend of mine found out that she suffered from a kidney disease. I didn't know so much about Kidney diseases and I was shocked when I discovered that my intimate friend had to deal with a serious health condition. I never heard my dear friend complaining about her illness, neither was she afraid of it. Yet, I was committed to help my friend lead an absolutely ordinary life and I accompanied her every time she would go to the hospital.

I had many conversations with other patients when my friend was seeing her doctor and many of them were on the verge of kidney failure. From the short time I spent with those patients, I learned that some of them used to work, but others gave up on living their normal lives and their only hope was dialysis once, twice or thrice a week. I was surprised that many patients didn't know what caused their illness and they were hoping that they had the ability to rewind time so that they eat healthy and never harm their kidneys.

And on this framework, I take pride in offering you this book and I dedicate my time and life to write it and offer it to all people suffering from kidney diseases in an attempt to help them cope with their kidney disease. It is never too late to cope with your kidney disease and to avoid dialysis, especially if you detect it on time. I don't claim I have the same medical knowledge as doctors and specialists, but through this book, I am offering you the best Renal Diet book that will be you your key guide to a healthy body and kidneys. Indeed, the cornerstone of healthy kidneys lies in the diet you follow.

Following a Renal diet can help limit the toxins and the waste in your body and can help your kidney function in a more effective way. So if you suffer from any kidney disease, don't feel discouraged and don't lose hope because a simple diet can change your life for the better forever. And remember that any tiny change in your meal plan can help prevent dialysis.

The "Cope with Kidney Disease and say good bye to Dialysis" diet Cookbook provides you with 70 delicious and healthy kidney-friendly meals accompanied by a detailed meal plan to help you organize better your meal every day. And even on a renal diet, you will still be able to enjoy incredibly delicious recipes with your friends, family and loved ones.

Chapter 1: Understanding the Renal Diet

Concept and etymology

Eating healthy and well is an important fact that can help you live longer and become stronger. And in some health conditions, a newly-adopted diet can be an indispensable solution and treatment that can help you feel better like you never felt before. In fact, not only the Renal Diet will make you feel better, but it can also prevent some serious complications of this unpleasant disease like high blood potassium, weight loss, fluid overload and bone disease.

The renal diet is an innovative diet that is mainly designed for people who suffer from a kidney disease. Wastes in the blood come from food and liquids that are consumed. People with kidney disease must adhere to a kidney diet to cut down on the amount of waste in their blood. Following a kidney diet may also bolster kidney function and delay total kidney failure.

For instance, a Renal Diet is characterised by being low in phosphorus, protein and sodium. Besides, a Renal Diet emphasizes the importance of limiting the intake of fluids and consuming proteins of high quality. Some types of kidney diets can also encourage lowering the consumption of calcium and potassium. And adopting any renal diet usually varies based on the condition of the patient and the stage of the kidney disease. Therefore, consulting a dietician is advised before adopting the renal diet.

And as it is known that fats and carbohydrates make the basic sources of the energy we need and we get from our food, the amount of milk, meat and eggs should be limited according to the patient's condition. Bread, cereals, pasta and rice should be limit to restricted quantities and amounts, in addition to some fruits and vegetables depending on the level of restricting phosphorus and potassium.

In a few words, a renal diet is a way of eating that can help you protect your kidneys' health from serious complications and from any further damage. And by following the renal diet, you can limit certain fluids and minerals. Simultaneously, adopting a renal diet, you should maintain the balance of proteins, vitamins and calories so that it won't overbuild up in your body.

And the renal diet is more effective if you are still in early stages of renal disease. Yet, as your disease can get worse, you should watch more what you eat and be more careful with what you put into your body because the ability of your kidneys to remove the wastes of your body starts declining. In fact, a renal diet can help you live healthier for a longer time. When the kidneys function in a normal way, your kidneys will be able to remove extra waste, water and any toxic substances from your body and turn it in urine. Only a balanced diet can improve the function of your affected kidneys. And following a renal diet can slow down any damage to your kidneys. And the meal plan you will find in this book can help you organise better your meals and maintain your food balanced.

Advantages of the renal diet

When the function of your kidneys starts slowing down, your entire lifestyle can be affected. Any disease that affects your kidneys can affect your nutritional status to a great extent and that happens mainly because kidneys play an important role in filtering toxic elements in your body. Eating too many unhealthy ingredients may result in the inability of the kidneys in excreting and hampers its function. So, following a renal diet is the safest solution to save our lies and prolong the function of our kidneys.

The renal diet has many benefits and enormous advantages that can help any kidney patient feel much better. Indeed, studies on people, who were diagnosed with different types of kidney diseases and who followed the renal diet, have proven that their symptoms improved. And in contrast, kidney patients who didn't follow any diet showed a considerable deterioration in their condition.

A renal diet is usually prescribed for patients whose kidneys start showing signs of malfunctioning. Doctors strongly recommend the renal diet for patients who have to undergo their dialysis. And here are some of the benefits of this diet:

1. The renal diet can improve the symptoms of kidney diseases.

The renal diet or what is also known as the kidney diet helps the patient feel better and helps relieve the symptoms of kidney diseases.

2. The renal diet helps slow down the worsening of the condition and prevents kidney failure

The renal diet has proven its ability in slowing down the development of kidney diseases and shows great results in slowing down kidney failure.

3. The renal diet helps decrease the level of phosphorus, protein and potassium

The levels of phosphorus, potassium and protein in our bodies make an important concern for all people, yet it is of a special concern in patients with kidney diseases. When the levels of those substances start being unbalanced, they can cause certain unbalanced illnesses. Thus, the renal diet can help patients to limit the level of proteins to the right amount, and it intervenes in maintaining the strength of the bones. Keeping the level of phosphorus low is also important to improve the health of the patient's heart.

4. Lowers the level of fluids

Kidney patients are usually advised to limit their fluid intake because of the inability of the kidneys to excrete high amounts of fluids within the body. Failure to comply with recommended fluid intake levels can result in annoying and painful swelling of the legs due to retain the fluids in certain parts of the body.

5. The renal diet can help reduce the risk of overweight and obesity

Healthy eating is the key to a healthy and fit body. Not only the renal diet can help reduce the risk of kidney diseases, but it can also manage a balanced weight.

6. The renal diet prevents diabetes, hyper-Lipidemia and hypertension

Adopting a renal diet is very effective in preventing obesity and all the diseases that can result from extra weight. Besides, this healthy renal diet can help avoid many serious health complications like cardiovascular diseases

7. The renal diet helps monitor the calorie intake

Consuming the needed amount of calories, no more no less, can help maintain a healthy body and weight. In fact, maintaining a moderate and balanced intake of calories can help prevent kidney failure.

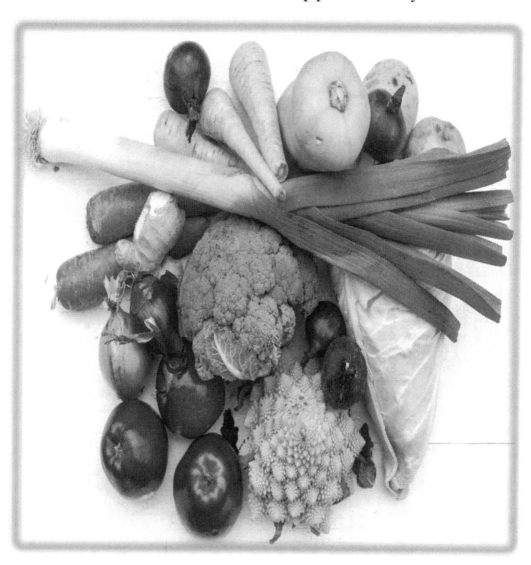

Controlling Your Potassium

Potassium is known as an element with a great importance for the role it plays in keeping the balance of water between the body fluids and its cells. All the foods we eat contain a certain quantity of potassium, but some ingredients contain high level of potassium that may endanger our health.

When kidneys function normally, they are able to remove the potassium from our blood through what we call urination. Yet, if kidneys start malfunctioning, it becomes quite impossible for kidneys to function properly and to remove extra potassium through urination. When potassium is not removed through urination it starts building up in the blood vessels, which can very extremely dangerous for the heart.

High levels of potassium can cause a certain irregularity in heart beats and are held for risking heart failure. And what is more dangerous about the potassium is that at high levels is that there no apparent symptoms that can warn us in advance.

And in order to manage your potassium level, you should check it on a regularly basis. Also, you should limit your daily intake of potassium to about 2000 mg per day

If you suspect high levels of potassium, you should avoid the following ingredients:

- Orange juices, Tomato juice
- Avocados and bananas
- Melon
- Cantaloupe Tomato
- White and red beans
- Black beans, Garbanzo beans and Lima Beans
- Split peas, lentils Split peas and baked Beans

Controlling Your Phosphorus

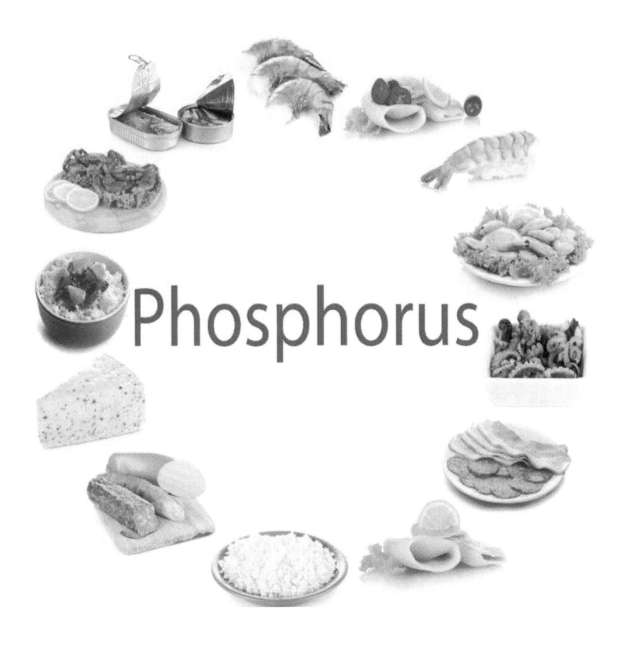

Phosphorus is a well-known mineral that the body can get rid of through the urine thanks to the help of healthy kidneys. However, if the kidneys are not functioning properly, phosphorus starts building up in the blood vessels and this may result in many serious health problems. The inability of kidneys to remove extra phosphorus from the body can cause several pains like, heart calcification, joint pain and leads to easily broken bones.

Phosphorus has always been related with the health of the bone and together with calcium bones are indispensable for maintaining strong bones. And in order to keep the level of phosphorus balanced in your body, you should carefully watch the foods you eat like meats, poultry, fish, beans, nuts and dairy products. Phosphorus is more likely to be found in animal foods and plant foods, yet our body absorbs the phosphorus we get from animal foods more than from plant foods.

The phosphorus that is added to certain foods is not as healthy as we can imagine because it comes in the form of preservatives and additives and it can be found in fast and junk foods. We might not know is that our body totally absorbs the phosphorus that we get from food additives. Hence, avoiding additives is the best way we can use to lower the intake phosphorus additives. You should always check the facts on the label of each food you buy and search for the "Phos" to be able to know which contain phosphorous more.

In order to maintain a balanced level of phosphorous and to keep it under control; here is what you should do:

Limit the consumption of foods like poultry, meats, fish and dairy

- Limit the intake of certain dairy products like yogurt and cheese; you should not exceed 4 oz per serving
- Avoid black beans, lima beans, red beans, garbanzo beans, white beans and black-eyed peas.
- Avoid unrefined, whole and dark grains.
- Stay away from refrigerator dough

- Avoid dried fruits and vegetables
- Avoid chocolate
- Try to limit the intake of dark colored sodas
- Make sure to take your phosphate binders with your snacks and meals.
- Don't forget to take your phosphate binders with meals and snacks.
- The renal diet limits the intake of phosphorus to 1000mg per day

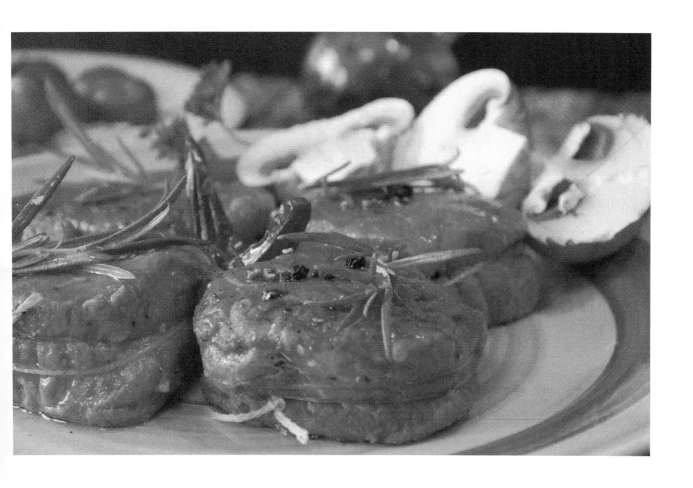

Controlling your Protein

Protein makes an essential element of our growth and it plays an important role in maintaining our body mass. Besides, proteins can help us fight any infection that can threaten our bodies. And while proteins are very important for our health, an excessive consumption may lead to undesirable and even threatening results. In fact, eating more than your body needs of proteins can hasten the deterioration of your kidneys.

Therefore, maintaining a moderate and balanced intake of proteins can keep your body healthy and it even can prevent kidney failure. Furthermore, when your kidneys are not able to function very well; they start leaking protein into your urine and this can lead to many unpleasant side effects like a change in taste, loss of appetite, nausea and even fatigue.

In a few words, protein is very important for the growth and the maintenance of our health and it is substantial in healing wounds, fighting all infections and providing our body with the energy it needs. Nevertheless, it's substantial to keep the level of proteins in our bodies balanced.

To make sure that our kidneys are not stressed by the proteins we eat, we should make sure to consume high-quality proteins. And we should make sure that we eat about 7 to 8 Oz of protein per day. 1 Egg equals 1 Oz of protein.

The foods that are high in protein include pork, beef, turkey, veal; chicken and eggs.

Controlling Your Sodium

Sodium, salt or sodium chloride is an ingredient that is used almost in every meal. In fact, salt is, by far, one of the most used ingredients on earth. And it is sodium that regulates the water level in or bodies.

We don't usually need any extra quantity of salt in our body; however the majority of people love salty food. But our desire for salt is toxic as any excessive use of this ingredient can cause a fluid retention in our bodies. Besides, an excessive use of salt can expand the volume of your blood, which can lead to swelling and high blood pressure. Moreover, consuming huge quantities of salt can lead to an excessive thirst.

In order o be able to give up on salt, try cooking with spices and herbs to add more flavour to your foods instead of using salt. And believe it or not, the less salt you use, the less you will feel craving for it; it is rather like an addiction.

Some people don't even notice that their foods are not prepared with salt when they eat at restaurants. And here are some steps that can help you limit sodium intake in a short time:

- Avoid the use of any type of table salt or any other ingredient that end with 'salt'
- Avoid any salt substitutes that may contain potassium
- Avoid any salty meats like ham, bacon, lunch meat and hot dogs
- Avoid any sort of salty snacks like nuts, cheese curls, chips and crackers
- Avoid all frozen dinners, instant noodles and canned soups
- Try not to use pickles, bottled sauces and olives

Controlling Your Fluid Intake

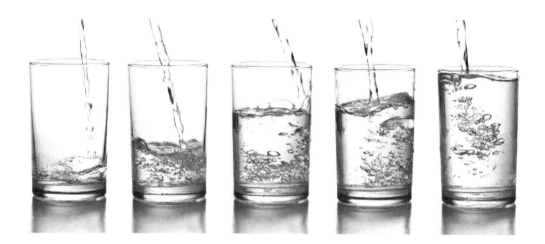

When your kidneys function properly, they are able to get rid of the fluids that enter our body. However, when our kidneys are not working properly and, our body might not be able to get rid of the fluids as it used to. The buildup of fluids in our body can lead to swelling, high blood pressure and even shortness of breath.

Therefore, we should limit our intake of fluids and we should keep it under control so that we can avoid dialysis at a certain step. There are many foods that are high in water like ice cream, sauces, rice pudding, gravy and custard. You should cut down on some food packed with water and avoid some other foods as well. Moreover, people who suffer from kidney diseases and who consume high levels of fluids may experience a pressure on the heart and the lungs.

And here are some tips with which you can restrict the intake of fluids:

1. Use 1 cup or glass in order to divide, your fluid intake per day. You can also write a record of your fluid intake.

2. Always avoid any type of salty food and never add extra salt to your meals.
3. Avoid processed meats, fast foods and canned foods
4. You can add lemon juice to the water you want to drink instead
5. You can rinse your mouth with a mouthwash from time to time
6. Avoid overheating
7. Maintain your blood sugar at a balanced level

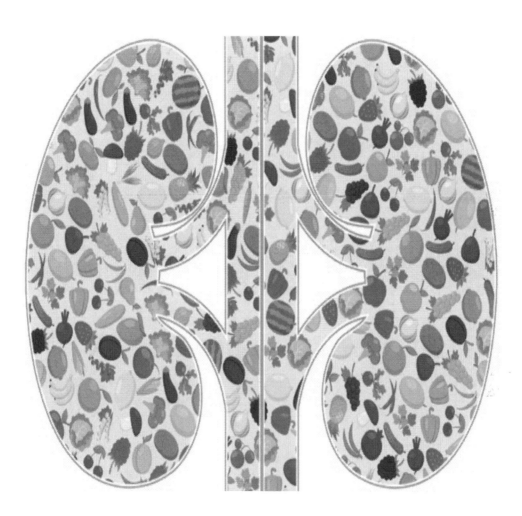

What to Eat and what not to eat on a renal diet

We eat different types of food so that we can get the energy our body needs to walk, work and do the different activities we love to. Yet, we should know that what we eat affects our health in different ways. When we have a special condition like kidney diseases, we should follow the best diet that can protect our kidneys from any further damage, which is the renal diet. And here is a list of what to eat and what not to eat on a renal diet:

What to Eat on a Renal Diet

Fruits

- Peaches
- Apples
- Strawberries
- Nectarines
- Celery
- Grapes
- Sweet bell peppers
- Spinach
- Hot peppers
- Cucumbers
- Kale, collard greens
- Cherry tomatoes
- Potatoes
- Imported snap peas
- Applesauce
- Apple, with its skin
- Apricots
- Applesauce

- Fresh or frozen blueberries
- Blackberries
- Boysenberries
- Cherries
- Casaba melon
- Fresh coconut
- Cranberries
- Crabapples
- Red, black or white currants
- Fruit cocktails
- Figs
- Grapefruit
- Gooseberries
- *Some people may be having some medication that shouldn't be taken with grapefruit

- Kumquat
- Grape
- Lime
- Lemon
- Frozen Loganberries
- Lychees
- Longans
- Maraschino cherries
- Passion fruit
- Mandarin orange
- Fresh pear
- American Persimmon

- Plums
- Pineapple
- Pomegranate (Always make sure to eat in small amount because it is high in potassium)
- Quince
- Prickly pear
- Fresh Rambutan
- Strawberries
- Rhubarb
- Watermelon

FOR THE CEREALS

- Puffed wheat
- Puffed Rice
- Shredded Wheat

- Rolled oats
- Regular Instant Oatmeal

Starches:

- Couscous
- Barley
- Pasta

- Brown or white rice
- Rice noodles
- White bread

Vegetables

- Raw Arugula
- Alfalfa sprouts

- Cooked not canned asparagus
- Canned Bamboo shoots

- Green bean sprouts
- Green bean
- Yellow beans
- Canned, non-pickled Beets
- Balsam pear or Bitter melon
- Cooked broccoli
- Green cabbage
- Napa Cabbage
- Red Cabbage
- Savoy Cabbage
- Cauliflower
- Fresh celery
- Celery root or Celeriac
- Fresh or frozen corn
- Cooked chayote
- Dandelion greens
- Endive
- Eggplant
- Fresh Fennel bulb
- Chinese broccoli, Gari lan
- Moo qua or fuzzy squash
- Canned grape leaves
- Raw Jicama
- Cooked Kale
- Lettuce
- Leeks
- Fresh or canned; but not cooked Mushrooms
- Shitake Mushrooms
- Enoki Mushrooms
- Frozen cooked mustard greens
- Cooked Nopales or cactus leaves
- Okra
- Onions
- Carrots and peas
- Green peas
- Red, yellow, green or orange peppers
- Hot chili, jalapeno peppers or hot chili
- Canned pumpkin
- Raw Radicchio
- Kelp and raw seaweed
- Nori seaweed
- Raw wakame seaweed wakame
- Raw shallots
- Cooked snow peas
- Spinach
- Cooked crookneck squash
- Cooked scallop squash
- Cooked spaghetti squash
- Raw zucchini
- Raw tomatillos
- Turnip
- Cooked, turnip greens
- Canned water chestnuts
- Raw watercress
- Cooked winter melon

Meat:

- Chicken
- Beef
- Duck
- Fresh types of eggs
- Omega pro eggs
- Egg Beaters
- Low in phosphorous egg whites
- Fresh fish
- Canned salmon without added phosphorus
- Low sodium tuna
- Lamb
- Game meat
- Seafood
- Pork
- Turkey
- Tofu
- Veal

Cheeses:

- Hard brick cheese
- Brie cheese
- Camembert cheese
- Low phosphorus cream cheese
- Soft goat cheese
- Coffee cream
- Ricotta cheese

Dairy products:

- No more than 1 cup of milk per day
- Low in phosphorus sour cream
- Frozen plain fruit
- Greek yogurt
- Low in phosphorus whipped cream
- Dairy alternative products
- Unsweetened vanilla

Drinks and juices

- Cranberry juice
- Blueberry Watermelon

- Mango juice
- Pink Grapefruit juice
- Homemade lemonade
- Strawberry juice
- Wild Berry juice

It is recommended to eat food ingredients that are usually close to nature like vegetables, fruits, peas and seeds. But make sure to avoid all types of foods that come in jars, boxes and that use preservatives and additives.

What Not to Eat on a Renal Diet

Here is the list of ingredients you should avoid in a renal diet:

- Pancake mixes or Baking mixes
- Crackers
- Canned stews and soups
- Canned vegetables
- Soy sauce and ketchup
- Chips, cheese puffs and pretzels
- Ramen noodles
- Flavored Rice or pasta
- Pickles foods
- Olives
- Frozen dinners
- Pickled foods, olives
- Processed meats like hot dogs and deli meats
- Vegetables and tomato juices
- Spaghetti sauce
- Avocados
- Bananas
- Beets and beet greens
- Carrot juice
- Clams
- Peas
- Chickpeas peas
- Soybeans
- Lentils
- Acorn hard squash
- Mangos
- Jerusalem artichokes
- Melons

- Molasses
- Salted Nuts
- Milk
- Molasses
- Parsnips
- Sweet potatoes and potatoes
- Spinach
- Tomato products and tomatoes
- Yogurt
- Fluids

Starches and sweets

- Corn and corn products
- Candy
- Peas and lentils
- Ice cream
- Plantains
- Wheat products including wheat bread, wheat bagels, cereal, cakes and crackers have to be limited
- White rice
- Some vegetables contain high level of phosphorus, so you should limit the following ingredients to 1 cup per week:
  - ➤ Greens, dried beans, mushrooms, Brussels sprouts and broccoli,
- Certain types of cereals like wheat cereals, granola, oatmeal and bran should be limited to 1serving per week.
- Whole grain bread is not allowed on a renal diet
- Beer is forbidden on renal diet.

> ➤ **Note:**

Some foods like squash and potatoes need to be cut into small dices or cubes in order to reduce the level of potassium in it. You should bring the small cubes to a boil; then drain it and add fresh water; then boil again. It may be quite surprising; but shellfish can harm your kidneys; so make sure to stay away from shellfish and include some antioxidants in your meal plan.

The Disadvantages of Fast Food for the Renal Patient

The renal diet was developed in order to compensate the low functioning of the kidneys. And the risks of not following a renal diet are much greater than the risk of following it. Yet, adopting a renal diet can, sometimes, have some risks.

For instance, the renal diet can cause a health condition called Hyponatremia and that condition takes occurs when the level of fluids, especially water and that of sodium are out of control. When the levels of potassium and sodium become severely low, the patient can show some symptoms of a dangerous and urgent emergency that needs immediate intervention.

When you adopt a renal diet, it can be very helpful for you to read the labels and the nutrition facts of each food product you purchase.

Low levels of sodium, potassium and fluids can cause unexplainable seizures, a coma or a sudden loss of consciousness. You can predict this condition with the help of certain symptoms like:

- Excessive weakness
- Low energy or fatigue
- Nausea
- Vomiting
- Headache
- Spasms or muscle cramps

- Irritability

So to avoid the risks of a renal diet, you should keep your food balanced; you should also keep the levels of intake of potassium, fluids, sodium and protein under control. And in addition to the renal diet, you should also take your medicines, if you have any, on time, it is also recommended to ask for the help of a nutritionist and to consult your Nephrologist to keep your health under control.

Meal Plan Tips

The Renal diet emphasizes that healthy food is the secret to healthy kidneys; it may also prevent dialysis at a certain point of our lives. This diet stresses out the importance of eating various foods and ingredients. And adopting a renal diet doesn't mean to give up on your favourite foods, but it teaches you to eat everything in moderation. And here are some tips you can follow when adopting the renal diet:

- Make sure to remove the skin of any poultry you are going to use
- Always avoid using table salts and oil
- Make sure not to eat fried noodles and opt rather for soup noodles
- Don't use packaged drinks with added sugar and choose healthier drinks
- Drink plain water instead of sweet drinks
- Cut down the consumption of fried meals and avoid high fat dishes to once or twice a week

- Reduce the consumption of fast foods
- Try not to add cheese to your spaghetti or pizza
- Cook brown rice instead of white rice
- Reduce the amount of seasoning in your meals
- Always use low fat cooking methods like boiling your food, steaming it, grilling or stir frying with as less oil as possible
- Enrich the flavours of your meals by using spices, herbs, vinegar or lemon juice
- Use healthy fats for cooking like coconut coil
- Use whole-meal noodle or brown rice
- When shopping, make sure to use ingredients with healthier nutrition labels
- Slow down when you eat; don't eat too quickly; it is very unhealthy to do that
- Do never eat when you feel full
- Always make sure to eat high proteins in main dishes like meat, fish and eggs
- Avoid eating nuts, peanut butter and seeds
- Choose cabbage and broccoli over asparagus and potatoes

Renal Diet Main FAQ

At the beginning of each new diet and life journey, many people ask so many questions before they make their final decision to start the diet. Being empowered with the required knowledge can help you understand better how any diet can affect your health and enables you to take the right and healthiest food choices. And to help you discover more information about the renal diet, here are a few of the main Frequent Asked Question you may ask before adopting the renal diet:

1. Who needs to adopt a renal diet?

Any person who is diagnosed with a kidney disease at any certain stage is advised to start making vital, immediate dietary changes. And the sooner you change your diet, the better. Indeed, the earlier you adopt a renal diet, the easier is to control the progression of your disease. In some cases, you can even save yourself from a dialysis.

2. How important is the renal diet for a kidney disease?

Adopting a specific diet can be the safest and easiest treatment for your kidney disease. For instance, even before taking medicines, changing the dietary habits can contribute to prevent your condition from worsening. In some cases, the renal diet can stop your disease completely.

3. What are the most important ingredients that renal diet restricts?

Salt or sodium is known for being one of the most important ingredients that the renal diet prohibits its use. This ingredient, although simple, can badly and strongly affect your body and especially the kidneys. Any excess of sodium can't be easily filtered because of the failing condition of the kidneys. A large build up of sodium can cause catastrophic results on your body.

Potassium and Phosphorus are also prohibited for kidney patients depending on the stage of kidney disease.

4. What are the best foods for a kidney patient?

The best foods for a renal patient are the foods that are, particularly, high in vitamins and low in sodium. Garlic, onion, red berries, apples and red bell pepper diet are foods that are low in sodium and high in vitamins and nutrients that can help your body rather than hurt it. Onions, garlic, bell peppers, red berries, and apples make great choices as best foods for kidney patients.

5. What is the worst food ingredient for a kidney patient?

Salty foods like crackers, chips and all salted foods make the worse of foods for kidney patients. Moreover, canned foods are also packed with sodium; which can worsen the condition of kidney patients. Highly processed foods are not an exception too.

6. How much sodium a person on renal diet should take?

A healthy renal diet should include no more than about 1500 to 2000mg of sodium per day.

7. What are the alternatives that can substitute salt in a renal diet?

There are certain types of spices and other ingredients that can substitute salt. You can use the Allspice, the basil, the bay leaf, the caraway, the cardamom, the curry, the dill, the ginger, the rosemary, the thyme, the sage, and the tarragon. You can also use vinegar and lemon juice in small quantities to give your dish the balance and to preserve the flavour you are used to.

> **Note:**

If you have any doubts and you have more questions, you can ask a nutritionist for the list of foods you should eat and to talk with your healthcare professional to avoid any problems.

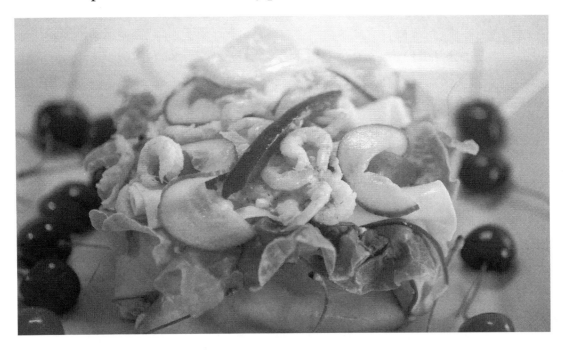

Chapter 2: Breakfast Recipes

Eggs in hole

(Prep time: 5 Mins|Cook Time: 10 Mins| Servings: 4)

Ingredients

- 4 Large eggs
- 4 Slices of white bread
- 4 tsp of margarine
- 1 tsp of Tabasco sauce

Instructions

1. Cut a hole in the centre of each bread slice with a small cup
2. Melt the margarine in a medium frying pan; then place the bread slices in your pan; make sure to turn the slices of bread to avoid burning it
3. Lightly coat both the sides of the bread with the margarine.
4. Cook on a medium high heat for about 1 to 2 minutes
5. Turn the cooked bread slices over; then break one large egg right into the centre of the hole in the bread slices
6. Cook for about 2 to 3 minutes or until the eggs are done
7. Toast your obtained bread circles and serve it with the eggs

Nutrition Information

Calories: 195, Fats: 10g, Carbs : 8g, Fiber : 2.1g, Potassium: 93mg, Sodium: 70mg, Phosphorous: 12mg, Protein 18 g

Kidney-friendly French toast

(Prep time: 5 Mins|Cook Time: 25 Mins| Servings: 6)

Ingredients

- 3 Large omega-3 eggs
- 3/4 Cup of almond milk
- 1 tablespoon of stevia
- 1 teaspoon of unsweetened vanilla
- ½ teaspoon of cinnamon
- 6 Slices of diagonally cut bread of 1 inch of thickness
- 1 tablespoon of margarine

Instructions

1. Beat the eggs with the milk, the stevia, the cinnamon and the vanilla in a large bowl
2. Soak the bread into the mixture of the eggs until it becomes smooth
3. Heat the margarine in a skillet and cook the bread over a medium high heat; make sure to flip from time to time for about 12 minutes per side
4. Serve your French toast and enjoy its taste!

Nutrition Information

Calories: 230, Fats : 14g, Carbs : 11g, Fiber : 2g, Potassium: 85mg, Sodium: 65mg, Phosphorus: 10mg, Protein 15 g

Fruit and rolled oat Pancakes

(Prep time: 10 Mins|Cook Time: 10 Mins| Servings: 5)

Ingredients

- ½ Cup of rolled oats
- 1 Cup of almond flour
- 8-oz of fruit cocktails
- ½ Cup of non-dairy creamer
- ½ teaspoon of unsalted phosphorus-free baking powder
- 1 Large omega-3 egg
- 1 tablespoon of margarine

Instructions

1. Combine all your ingredients together in a large bowl except for the margarine.
2. Melt the margarine in a large pan or skillet.
3. Pour the batter into the skillet; about ¼ cups per each pancake and cook it over a medium heat or until the pancakes become bubbly
4. Flip pancake with a spatula and cook it until it becomes gold
5. Serve and enjoy your pancakes!

Nutrition Information

Calories: 126, Fats : 6g, Carbs : 10.9g, Fiber : 0.7g, Potassium: 100mg, Sodium: 98mg, Phosphorous: 101mg, Protein 7 g

Deviled eggs

(Prep time: 7 Mins|Cook Time: 12 Mins| Servings: 8)

Ingredients

- 1 Pinch of paprika
- 1 Pinch of ground black pepper
- 2 tbsp of vegan mayonnaise
- ½ tsp of dry mustard
- ½ tsp of vinegar
- 1 tbsp of finely chopped onion
- 4 Omega-3 hard boiled eggs

Instructions

1. Start by cutting the eggs into halves lengthwise; then remove the yolk and mash it with a fork
2. Combine the yolk with the rest of the ingredients in a large bowl except for the paprika
3. Refill the egg whites with the mixed yolks; then sprinkle with a little bit of paprika
4. Serve and enjoy your breakfast!

Nutrition Information

Calories: 136, Fats : 11g, Carbs : 2g, Fiber : 0.3g, Potassium: 37mg, Sodium: 94mg, Phosphorous: 92mg, Protein 7 g

Omelet with onion and apple

(Prep time: 10 Mins| Cook Time: 20 Mins| Servings: 3)

Ingredients

- 3 large omega-3 eggs
- ¼ Cup of 1% low fat milk
- 1 tablespoon of water
- 1/8 teaspoon of black pepper
- 1 tablespoon of almond butter
- ¾ cup of sweet onion
- 1 Apple

Instructions

1. Preheat your oven to a temperature of about 400° F.
2. Peel and core the apple; then thinly slice it and slice the onion as well
3. Beat the eggs with the milk, the water and the pepper in a medium bowl and set it aside.
4. In a small oven-proof large skillet and over a medium high heat, melt the almond butter Add the onion and the apple to the skillet and sauté the ingredients for about 5 to 6 minutes
5. Spread out the apple mixture and the onion in your skillet
6. Pour the egg mixture in an even way in your skillet and cook over a medium high heat for a couple of minutes
7. Transfer the skillet to the oven and bake your omelette for about 10 minutes Remove the skillet from the oven and set it aside to cool for a few minutes
8. Serve and enjoy your omelette.

Nutrition Information

Calories: 215, Fats : 13g, Carbs : 11.6g, Fiber : 3.2g, Potassium: 99mg, Sodium: 91mg, Phosphorous: 89mg, Protein 13 g

Breakfast Pork casserole

(Prep time: 5 Mins| Cook Time: 60 Mins| Servings: 9)

Ingredients

- 8 Oz of reduced-fat pork sausage
- 8 Ounces of cream cheese
- 1 Cup of almond milk
- 4 Cubed slices of white bread
- 5 large omega-3 eggs
- ½ teaspoon of dry mustard
- ½ teaspoon of dried onion flakes

Instructions

1. Preheat your oven to a temperature of about 325 F°.
2. Crumble the pork sausage and cook it in a medium skillet over a medium high heat; then set it aside.
3. Toss all your ingredients together except for the bread in a blender
4. Add the cooked sausage to your mixture
5. Place the bread pieces in a casserole dish; then pour the sausage mixture over the bread
6. Bake your dish for about 55 minutes
7. Cut your baked sausage casserole breakfast into about 9 portions
8. Serve and enjoy your breakfast!

Nutrition Information

Calories: 224, Fats : 16g, Carbs : 9g, Fiber : 0.4g, Potassium: 101mg, Sodium: 115mg, Phosphorous: 98mg, Protein 11 g

Pepper Quiche

(Prep time: 5 Mins|Cook Time: 55 Mins| Servings: 7)

Ingredients

- 1 Tablespoon of margarine
- 1 Sliced green pepper
- 1 Sliced sweet red pepper
- 1 Sweet sliced yellow pepper
- 1 Cup of low cholesterol egg substitute
- 1/2 Cup of liquid non-dairy creamer
- ½ Cup of water
- ½ teaspoon of basil
- 1/8 teaspoon of cayenne
- 1 Pinch of pepper
- 1 Unbaked pie shell of 9 inches

Instructions

1. In a large skillet and over a medium high heat, sauté the pepper in the margarine until it becomes soft
2. Combine the egg substitute with the creamer, the water, the basil and the cayenne
3. Spoon the peppers into the centre of the unbaked pie shell; then pour the egg mixture over the peppers and bake in the oven at a temperature of about 375°F for about 50 to 55 minutes and set aside for about 10 minutes until it cools down
4. Slice your quiche; then serve and enjoy its delicious taste!

Nutrition Information

Calories: 159, Fats : 10.5g, Carbs : 11g, Fiber : 1.9g, Potassium: 163mg, Sodium: 222mg, Phosphorous: 50mg, Protein 5g

Egg Benedict

(Prep time: 10 Mins|Cook Time: 20 Mins| Servings: 4)

Ingredients

- 4 Ounces of sliced Canadian bacon
- 3 Cups of water
- 3 Cups of English muffins
- 2 Muffins
- 1 Tablespoon of vinegar
- 4 Omega-3 Eggs
- ½ Cup of unsalted butter
- 3 Egg yolks
- 1 Dash of cayenne pepper
- 1 Pinch of paprika
- 1 Tablespoon of lemon juice

Instructions

1. De-mineralize the Canadian bacon by placing it in 2 cups of boiling water for about 5 minutes.
2. Remove the Canadian bacon with a slotted spoon and set it right on top of several paper towels so that it can help it absorb the moisture.
3. Now, slice the English muffins into half and toast it on both sides
4. Cut the Canadian bacon into half; then place it on top of each of the toasted muffin halves
5. Combine the vinegar with 1 cup of water in a large heavy skillet
6. Bring the ingredients to a boil; then reduce the heat
7. Break the eggs one by one; then carefully lip it into the water and poach your eggs
8. Cover the skillet with a lid and let simmer for about 5 minutes

9. Remove the eggs with a slotted spoon and place it on top of the bacon and the muffins and set it aside to keep it warm
10. Melt the butter and beat the egg yolks over a high heat; then quickly add in the egg yolks over a very light heat
11. Add in the melted butter, the paprika and the cayenne pepper.
12. Beat in the lemon juice until your ingredients become thick
13. Remove from the heat; then pour over the English muffins
14. Serve and enjoy your breakfast!

Nutrition Information

Calories: 307, Fats : 22g, Carbs : 11.2g, Fiber : 1.05g, Potassium: 174mg, Sodium: 345mg, Phosphorous: 214mg, Protein 16g

Waffles with cocoa powder

(Prep time: 7 Mins|Cook Time: 15 Mins| Servings: 5)

Ingredients

- 5 tablespoons of unsweetened cocoa powder
- 5 tablespoons of olive oil
- 1 tablespoon of ground flax
- ½ teaspoon of Splenda
- ¼ cup of fat free milk
- ½ Cup of egg white

Instructions

1. Mix all your ingredients together in a bowl and mix very well
2. Once your mixture is smooth, add 1 spoonful of the dough to the waffle iron and cook for a few minutes
3. Repeat the same process with the remaining dough until you finish it all
4. Top your waffles with chopped fruits, but never use bananas
5. Serve and enjoy your waffles!

Nutrition Information

Calories: 185, Fats : 15g, Carbs : 6.7g, Fiber : 0.9g, Potassium: 108mg, Sodium: 79mg, Phosphorous: 96mg, Protein 5.3g

Cauliflower and broccoli gratin

(Prep time: 10 Mins|Cook Time: 30 Mins| Servings: 4)

Ingredients

- 1 Package of 16 oz of cauliflower and broccoli
- ½ Cup of reduced Fat Mayonnaise
- ½ Cup of shredded unsalted mozzarella cheese
- 1/2 cup of shredded cheddar cheese
- ½ Cup of sliced green onions
- 3 small onions
- 1 Minced garlic clove
- 1 Tablespoon of Dijon mustard
- 1/8 Teaspoon of cayenne pepper or ground red pepper
- 1/8 teaspoon of Italian seasoned white breadcrumbs
- ¼ tablespoons of paprika

Instructions

1. Preheat your oven to a temperature of about 350 degrees.
2. Arrange the broccoli and cauliflower florets in a microwave steamer for about 4 to 5 minutes
3. Lightly grease a baking dish of about 2 quarts; then arrange the florets in its bottom
4. Add the mayonnaise, the mozzarella cheese, the Parmesan cheese, the green onions, the garlic, the mustard and the red pepper to the baking dish
5. Sprinkle with the breadcrumbs and the paprika.
6. Bake for about 20 to 25 minutes in the oven
7. Serve and enjoy your breakfast!

Nutrition Information

Calories: 150, Fats: 13g, Carbs: 5.2g, Fiber: 1.1g, Potassium: 200mg, Sodium: 19mg, Phosphorous: 90mg, Protein 3g

Wheat Berry bowl

(Prep time: 10Mins|Cook Time: 20 Mins| Servings: 2)

Ingredients

- ½ cups of uncooked wheat berries
- 1 Medium fresh pear
- 1 tablespoon of almond butter
- ½ cup of fresh cranberries
- 2 tablespoons of crystallized ginger
- 1 teaspoons of fresh orange zest
- 2 tablespoons of stevia
- ½ teaspoon of cinnamon

Instructions

1. To cook the wheat berries, bring about 1 and 1/2 cups of water and about ½ cup of wheat berries to boil.
2. Turn down the heat to a simmer and cover the pan with a lid
3. Check you mixture for doneness; then thinly slice the pear and cook for about 15 minutes and make sure to check for every 5 minutes
4. Heat the butter in a sauté pan and add the pear slices; then cook until your mixture becomes tender.
5. Add the cranberries and the chopped crystallized ginger to the pears and cook for about 4 minutes
6. Add the cooked wheat berries, the orange zest, the stevia and the cinnamon
7. Stir for a few minutes
8. Serve and enjoy your breakfast!

Nutrition Information

Calories: 161, Fats : 12g, Carbs : 9g, Fiber : 0.44g, Potassium: 235mg, Sodium: 139.5mg, Phosphorous: 93mg, Protein 4.2g

Unsalted, Breakfast tortillas

(Prep time: 5 Mins|Cook Time: 10 Mins| Servings: 4)

Ingredients

- 4 large beaten eggs
- 4 small, unsalted tortillas
- 2 teaspoons of olive oil
- 1 tablespoon of Mrs. Dash® Original Blend
- ¼ Cup of shredded cheddar cheese
- 1 Dash of Tabasco
- 1 Pinch of salt
- 1 Pinch of ground black pepper

Instructions

1. Heat the oil in a large skillet over a medium high heat and once the oil heats up; add in the original blend with the beaten eggs
2. Cook the beaten eggs for about 2 minutes; make sure to stir from time to time to prevent sticking and burning
3. Add in the cheese and keep stirring
4. Put a spoonful of the mixture over the tortillas; then roll it up and serve it with the ketchup
5. Enjoy your breakfast!

Nutrition Information

Calories: 115.8, Fats : 6g, Carbs : 11.7g, Fiber : 05g, Potassium: 67.2mg, Sodium: 203mg, Phosphorous: 87.4mg, Protein 3.6g

Breakfast Couscous

(Prep time: 8 Mins|Cook Time: 35 Mins| Servings: 3-4)

Ingredients

- 1 and ¾ cups of water
- 2 tablespoons of old fashioned uncooked grits
- 1 tablespoon of uncooked bulgur
- 1 tablespoon of uncooked roasted whole buckwheat
- 1 tablespoon of uncooked steel-cut oats
- 3 tablespoons of plain uncooked couscous

Instructions

1. Boil the water in a covered pot
2. Add in the grits and briefly cook
3. Add the bulgur, the buckwheat, and the oats; then stir briefly.
4. Reduce the heat to a simmer and spray the surface with non-stick spray
5. Cover the pot and let simmer for about 25 minutes.
6. Remove the pot from the burner and stir in the couscous.
7. Let your pot stand covered for about 8 minutes
8. Serve and enjoy your breakfast!

Nutrition Information

Calories: 135, Fats : 5g, Carbs : 12g, Fiber : 1.9g, Potassium: 90mg, Sodium: 66mg, Phosphorous: 91mg, Protein 10g

Breakfast Custard

(Prep time: 5 Mins|Cook Time: 10 Mins| Servings: 3)

Ingredients

- 1/3 Cup of quick-cooking oatmeal
- 1 large omega-3 egg
- ½ Cup of almond milk
- ¼ teaspoon of cinnamon
- ½ Apple

Instructions

1. Core the apple; then cut the apple into halves
2. Combine the oats, the egg and the almond milk into a large mug; then stir your ingredients with a fork
3. Add the cinnamon and the apple and stir until your ingredients are fully mixture
4. Cook your batter in a microwave on a high heat for about 2 minutes.
5. Fluff the mixture with the help of a fork; then cook for about 50 seconds
6. You can add more milk if the mixture is too thick!

Nutrition Information

Calories: 156, Fats: 8g, Carbs: 9g, Fiber: 2.3g, Potassium: 265mg, Sodium: 163mg, Phosphorous: 240mg, Protein 11g

Breakfast Berry bowl

(Prep time: 10Mins|Cook Time: 20 Mins| Servings: 2)

Ingredients

- ½ cups of uncooked wheat berries
- 1 Medium fresh pear
- 1 tablespoon of almond butter
- ½ cup of fresh cranberries
- 2 tablespoons of crystallized ginger
- 1 teaspoons of fresh orange zest
- 2 tablespoons of stevia
- ½ teaspoon of cinnamon

Instructions

9. To cook the wheat berries, bring about 1 and 1/2 cups of water and about ½ cup of wheat berries to boil.
10. Turn down the heat to a simmer and cover the pan with a lid
11. Check you mixture for doneness; then thinly slice the pear and cook for about 15 minutes and make sure to check for every 5 minutes
12. Heat the butter in a sauté pan and add the pear slices; then cook until your mixture becomes tender.
13. Add the cranberries and the chopped crystallized ginger to the pears and cook for about 4 minutes
14. Add the cooked wheat berries, the orange zest, the stevia and the cinnamon
15. Stir for a few minutes
16. Serve and enjoy your breakfast!

Nutrition Information

Calories: 164, Fats: 13g, Carbs: 8.5g, Fiber: 0.7g, Potassium: 200mg, Sodium: 19mg, Phosphorous: 90mg, Protein 3g

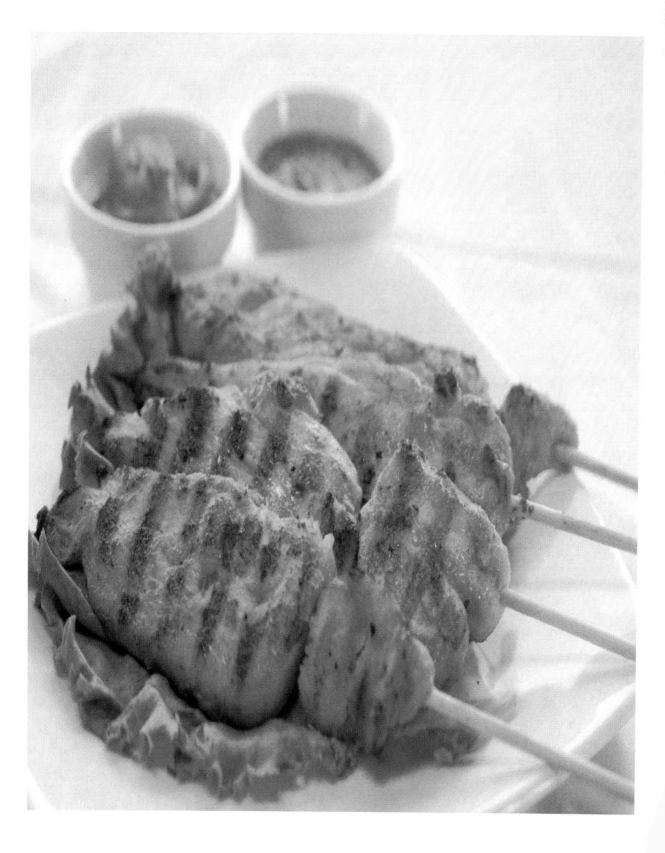

Chapter 3 Lunch Recipes

Pork chops with apple

(Prep time: 8 Mins|Cook Time: 78 Mins| Servings: 4)

Ingredients

- 2 Cored and sliced apples
- 2 Tablespoons of olive oil
- 4 Pork chops of about 6 oz with the centre cut
- ½ Cup of water
- 2 Teaspoon of stevia
- 2 Tablespoons of cider vinegar
- 1 Pinch of pepper

Instructions

1. Preheat your oven to about 325°F.
2. Heat the olive oil in a large skillet over a medium-high heat or until the oil starts shimmering
3. Add in the pork chops and brown each chop on both sides
4. Arrange the pork chops in the bottom of an oven-proof pan; then lay the apples right over the top
5. Deglaze the large skillet you have used by pouring ½ cup of water in it; then stir and remove all the bits of pork
6. Pour the mixture of the water and oil on top of the apples and the pork chops; then drizzle with the vinegar and add the stevia
7. Season with the pepper; then cover your dish and bake for about 30 minutes in the oven
8. Remove the cover of the dish and bake for about 40 additional minutes
9. Serve and enjoy your lunch!

Nutrition Information

Calories: 395, Fats: 22g, Carbs: 16g, Fiber: 1.4g, Potassium: 59mg, Sodium: 320mg, Phosphorous: 235mg, Protein 33g

Lamb with fruit sauce

(Prep time: 5 Mins|Cook Time: 10 Mins| Servings: 2)

Ingredients

- 1 Minced garlic clove
- 1 tsp of dry rosemary
- ½ tsp of Mrs Dash herb seasoning
- 2 lamb chops of about 12 Oz
- 2 Tablespoons of stevia
- 1 tsp of spicy brown mustard
- 1 tsp of grated orange peel
- 1 Tablespoon of water

Instructions

1. Mince the garlic and mix it with the rosemary and the herb seasoning
2. Spread the seasoning over the lamb; broil the lamb about 6 inches from the heat for about 5 minutes
3. Mix the marmalade, the mustard, and the orange peel with a little bit of water in a glass dish; then mix very well and microwave the mixture for about 1 minute
4. Spread the mixture over the lamb chops and broil it in the oven for about 1 minute
5. Serve and enjoy your lunch!

Nutrition Information

Calories: 397, Fats: 25g, Carbs: 9g, Fiber: 1.9g, Potassium: 292mg, Sodium: 255mg, Phosphorous: 155mg, Protein 34g

Slow Cooked chuck roast with onion

(Prep time: 10 Mins|Cook Time: 2 Hours| Servings: 4)

Ingredients

- 1 large white onion
- 2 Tablespoon of avocado oil
- 1 Tablespoon of dried basil
- 1 Tablespoon of garlic powder
- 1 Pinch of cayenne pepper
- 2 to 3 pounds of chuck roast

Instructions:

1. Spray your slow cooker with cooking spray
2. Thinly slice the onion and place it in your slow cooker
3. Sprinkle in the garlic powder, the cayenne pepper and the dried basil over the onion.
4. Turn on the slow cooker and cover it with lid; then cook for about ½ hour on High
5. Remove the lid and flip the meat; then replace the lid and cook for about 1 and ½ hours on low
6. When the time is up, turn off your slow cooker
7. Serve the meat in platter and top with onion
8. Enjoy your lunch!

Nutrition Information

Calories: 414, Fats: 21g, Carbs: 13g, Fiber: 1.7g, Potassium: 49mg, Sodium: 216mg, Phosphorous: 156mg, Protein 35g

Pork Tenderloin with cumin

(Prep time: 5 Mins|Cook Time: 45 Mins| Servings: 3)

Ingredients

- 2 Pounds of boneless pork loin roast
- 3 to 3 minced garlic cloves
- ½ tsp of ground black pepper
- 2 tsp of allspice
- 2 tsp of onion powder
- ½ tsp of cumin
- 2 Tablespoons of olive oil

Instructions:

1. Mix the minced garlic with the black pepper and the allspice in a small bowl
2. Rub the tenderloin with the spices, then place the meat in a large dish and refrigerate it for about 2 hours
3. Heat your oven to a temperature of about 350°F
4. Drizzle a baking pan with the oil; then place the tenderloin in the dish
5. Roast the tenderloin uncovered for about 45 minutes
6. Serve and enjoy your lunch!

Nutrition Information

Calories: 440, Fats: 27g, Carbs: 10.2g, Fiber: 2.1g, Potassium: 50mg, Sodium: 360mg, Phosphorous: 242mg, Protein 39g

Slow cooked chicken with lemon and oregano

(Prep time: 8 Mins|Cook Time: 8 Hours| Servings: 8)

Ingredients

- 1 Tablespoon of olive oil
- 2 Minced garlic cloves
- 1 tsp of oregano
- 2 Pounds of bone-in chicken breast
- 13 of reduced sodium chicken broth
- 3 Tablespoons of lemon juice

Instructions:

1. Heat the olive oil in a large skillet.
2. Add the garlic and the oregano to the skillet and cook for about 1 minute
3. Add the chicken breast and brown the chicken on all its sides
4. Add the browned chicken to a slow cooker and pour the broth over it; and cook on Low for about 6 to 8 hours
5. Add about 3 tablespoons of lemon juice in the last hour
6. Serve and enjoy your lunch!

Nutrition Information

Calories: 298, Fats: 18g, Carbs: 8g, Fiber: 1.1g, Potassium: 288mg, Sodium: 182mg, Phosphorous: 206mg, Protein 26g

Oven Baked Halibut

(Prep time: 5 Mins|Cook Time: 20 Mins| Servings: 3)

Ingredients

- 2 Skin-on halibut fillets of about 5oz
- 1 tsp of olive oil
- 1 Minced large garlic clove
- 2 tsp of lemon zest
- The juice of ½ a lemon
- 1 tbsp of chopped flat leaf parsley
- 1 Pinch of ground black pepper

Instructions:

1. Preheat your oven to a temperature of about 400°F.
2. Add the halibut to a large non-stick baking dish
3. Add the halibut with the skin down into the baking dish and drizzle it with oil
4. Top with the garlic, a little bit of parsley, the lemon zest and about 2 tbsp of lemon juice
5. Season your halibut with the pepper and bake for about 15 minutes
6. Pour the lemon juice over the halibut steak
7. Serve and enjoy your lunch!

Nutrition Information

Calories: 300, Fats: 16g, Carbs: 8.9g, Fiber: 0.6g, Potassium: 233mg, Sodium: 176mg, Phosphorous: 360mg, Protein 30g

Garlic Shrimp

(Prep time: 5 Mins|Cook Time: 10 Mins| Servings: 3)

Ingredients

- 1 Pound of shrimp in shells
- ½ Cup of melted, unsalted margarine,
- 2 Teaspoons of lemon juice
- 2 Tablespoons of chopped onion
- 1 Minced garlic clove
- 1/8 teaspoon of pepper
- 1 Tablespoon of chopped fresh parsley

Instructions:

1. Preheat your broiler; then wash the shrimp, peel it and dry it with clean paper towels
2. Pour the margarine in a baking pan; then add the lemon juice, the onion, the pepper and the garlic
3. Add in the shrimp and toss very well
4. Broil the shrimps for about 5 minutes; then flip the shrimps and broil for 5 additional minutes
5. Transfer the broiled shrimp to a serving dish
6. Sprinkle the shrimp with parsley
7. Serve and enjoy your dish!

Nutrition Information

Calories: 279, Fats: 19g, Carbs: 7.8g, Fiber: 1.3g, Potassium: 189mg, Sodium: 135mg, Phosphorous: 192mg, Protein 19g

Spicy fish with peppers

(Prep time: 10 Mins|Cook Time: 15 Mins| Servings: 4)

Ingredients

- 1 and ½ pounds of white fish fillets
- 1 teaspoon of garlic powder
- ½ teaspoon of lemon pepper
- 2 tablespoons of oil
- ½ Cup of low-sodium chicken broth
- ¼ Cup of no-salt-added tomato sauce
- 1 Teaspoon of capers
- ½ Cut into rings green pepper
- ½ Cut into rings medium red pepper

Instructions:

1. Cut the fish into piece of 4 inches each
2. Sprinkle the fish with lemon pepper and garlic powder
3. Cook the fish in hot oil in a large non-stick skillet over a medium heat for about 5 minutes; make sure to turn from time to time
4. Add the broth, the low sodium tomato sauce and the capers; then reduce the heat and cover the skillet with a lid
5. Let your ingredients simmer for about 10 minutes
6. Top with the pepper rings and cook for 5 additional minutes
7. Serve and enjoy your lunch!

Nutrition Information

Calories: 254, Fats: 13g, Carbs: 11g, Fiber: 1.7g, Potassium: 290mg, Sodium: 104mg, Phosphorous: 350mg, Protein 23g

Spicy Chicken Marsala

(Prep time: 7 Mins|Cook Time: 20 Mins| Servings: 3)

Ingredients

- ½ Cup of shallots
- 2 Cups of fresh mushrooms
- 5 Tablespoons of fresh parsley
- 4 Boneless and skinless chicken breasts
- ½ Cup of white flour
- 1 Cup of all-purpose white flour
- 2 tablespoons of olive oil
- 2 tablespoons of butter-olive oil blend spread
- 1/3 Cup of dry Marsala wine
- ¼ teaspoon of garlic powder
- 1/8 teaspoon of black pepper
- 2 Cups of cooked white rice

Instructions:

1. Slice the shallots and the mushrooms; then chop the parsley.
2. Coat the chicken with the flour. In a large non-stick skillet, cook the chicken in heated oil over a medium high heat for about 10 minutes and make sure to flip the chicken from time to time
3. Sauté the shallots, the mushrooms and about 4 tablespoons of parsley into olive oil and blend it over a medium heat for about 3 minutes
4. Add the Marsala wine, the garlic powder and the black pepper. Cook your mixture while stirring for about 2 minutes
5. Pour the sauce and the vegetables over the chicken.
6. Sprinkle with the remaining parsley.
7. Serve your lunch with about ½ cup of the cooked white rice!

Nutrition Information

Calories: 407, Fats: 25g, Carbs: 13.5g, Fiber: 3.2g, Potassium: 320mg, Sodium: 145mg, Phosphorous: 300mg, Protein 32g

Chicken Curry

(Prep time: 10 Mins|Cook Time: 9 Hours| Servings: 5)

Ingredients

- 2 to 3 boneless chicken breasts
- ¼ Cup of chopped green onions
- 1 can of 4 oz of diced green chilli peppers
- 2 Teaspoons of minced garlic
- 1 and 1/2 teaspoons of curry powder
- 1 Teaspoon of chili Powder
- 1 Teaspoon of cumin
- ½ Teaspoon of cinnamon
- 1 Teaspoon of lime juice
- 1 and 1/2 cups water
- 1 can or 7 oz of coconut milk
- 2 Cups of white cooked rice
- Chopped cilantro, for garnish

Instructions:

1. Combine the green onion with the chicken, the green chilli peppers, the garlic, the curry powder, the chilli powder, the cumin, the cinnamon, the lime juice, and the water in the bottom of a 6-qt slow cooker
2. Cover the slow cooker with a lid and cook your ingredients on Low for about 7 to 9 hours
3. After the cooking time ends up; shred the chicken with the help of a fork
4. Add in the coconut milk and cook on High for about 15 minutes
5. Top the chicken with cilantro; then serve your dish with rice
6. Enjoy your lunch!

Nutrition Information

Calories: 254, Fats: 18g, Carbs: 6g, Fiber: 1.6g, Potassium: 370mg, Sodium: 240mg, Phosphorous: 114mg, Protein 17g

Steak with onion

(Prep time: 5 Mins|Cook Time: 60 Mins| Servings: 7-8)

Ingredients:

- ¼ Cup of white flour
- 1/8 Teaspoon of ground black pepper
- 1 and ½ pounds of round steak of ¾ inch of thickness each
- 2 Tablespoons of oil
- 1 Cup of water
- 1 tablespoon of vinegar
- 1 Minced garlic clove
- 1 to 2 bay leaves
- ¼ teaspoon of crushed dried thyme
- 3 Sliced medium onions

Instructions:

1. Cut the steak into about 7 to 8 equal servings. Combine the flour and the pepper; then pound the ingredients all together into the meat.
2. Heat the oil in a large skillet over a medium high heat and brown the meat on both its sides
3. Remove the meat from the skillet and set it aside
4. Combine the water with the vinegar, the garlic, the bay leaf and the thyme in the skillet; then bring the mixture to a boil
5. Place the meat in the mixture and cover it with onion slices
6. Cover your ingredients and let simmer for about 55 to 60 minutes
7. Serve and enjoy your lunch!

Nutrition Information

Calories: 286, Fats: 18g, Carbs: 12g, Fiber: 2.25g, Potassium: 368mg, Sodium: 45mg, Phosphorous: 180mg, Protein 19g

Shrimp scampi

(Prep time: 4 Mins|Cook Time: 8 Mins| Servings: 3)

Ingredients:

- 1 Tablespoon of olive oil
- 1 Minced garlic clove
- ½ Pound of cleaned and peeled shrimp
- ¼ Cup of dry white wine
- 1 Tablespoon of lemon juice
- ½ teaspoon of basil
- 1 tablespoon of chopped fresh parsley
- 4 Oz of dry linguini

Instructions

1. Heat the oil in a large non-stick skillet; then add the garlic and the shrimp and cook while stirring for about 4 minutes
2. Add the wine, the lemon juice, the basil and the parsley
3. Cook for about 5 minutes longer; then boil the linguini in unsalted water for a few minutes
4. Drain the linguini; then top it with the shrimp
5. Serve and enjoy your lunch!

Nutrition Information

Calories: 340, Fats: 26g, Carbs: 11.3g, Fiber: 2.1g, Potassium: 189mg, Sodium: 85mg, Phosphorous: 167mg, Protein 15g

Chicken Paella

(Prep time: 5 Mins|Cook Time: 10 Mins| Servings: 8)

Ingredients:

- ½ Pound of skinned, boned and cut into pieces, chicken breasts
- 1/4 Cup of water
- 1 Can of 10-1/2 oz of low-sodium chicken broth
- ½ Pound of peeled and cleaned medium-size shrimp
- 1/2 Cup of frozen green pepper
- 1/3 cup of chopped red bell
- 1/3 cup of thinly sliced green onion
- 2 Minced garlic cloves
- 1/4 Teaspoon of pepper
- 1 Dash of ground saffron
- 1 Cup of uncooked instant white rice

Instructions:

1. Combine the first 3 ingredients in medium casserole and cover it with a lid; then microwave it for about 4 minutes
2. Stir in the shrimp and the following 6 ingredients; then cover and microwave the shrimp on a high heat for about 3 and ½ minutes
3. Stir in the rice; then cover and set aside for about 5 minutes
4. Serve and enjoy your paella!

Nutrition Information

Calories: 236, Fats: 11g, Carbs: 6g, Fiber: 1.2g, Potassium: 178mg, Sodium: 83mg, Phosphorous: 144mg, Protein 28g

Beef Kabobs with pepper

(Prep time: 5 Mins|Cook Time: 10 Mins| Servings: 8)

Ingredients:

- 1 Pound of beef sirloin
- ½ Cup of vinegar
- 2 tbsp of salad oil
- 1 Medium, chopped onion
- 2 tbsp of chopped fresh parsley
- ¼ tsp of black pepper
- 2 Cut into strips green peppers

Instructions

1. Trim the fat from the meat; then cut it into cubes of 1 and ½ inches each
2. Mix the vinegar, the oil, the onion, the parsley and the pepper in a bowl
3. Place the meat in the marinade and set it aside for about 2 hours; make sure to stir from time to time.
4. Remove the meat from the marinade and alternate it on skewers instead with green pepper
5. Brush the pepper with the marinade and broil for about 10 minutes 4 inches from the heat
6. Serve and enjoy your kabobs

Nutrition Information

Calories: 357, Fats: 24g, Carbs: 9g, Fiber: 2.3g, Potassium: 250mg, Sodium: 60mg, Phosphorous: 217mg, Protein 26g

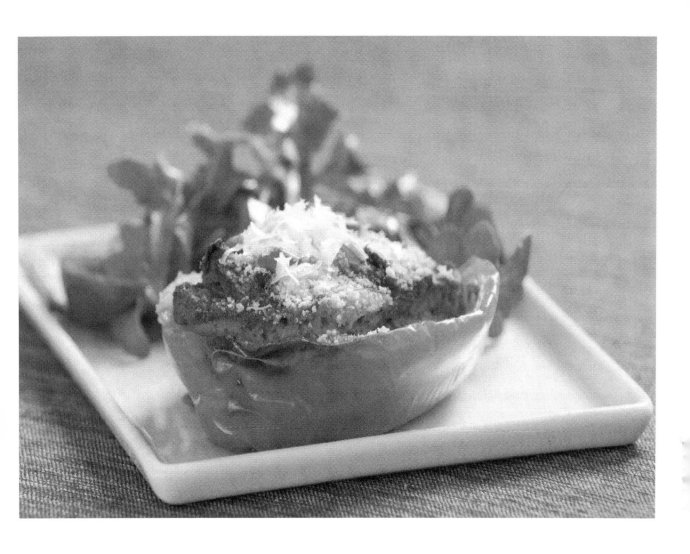

Chapter 4 Appetizer, snack or salad

Egg Rolls

(Prep time: 10 Mins| Cook Time: 30 Mins| Servings: 10)

Ingredients:

- 1 Pound of diced cooked chicken
- ½ Pound of bean sprouts
- ½ Pound of shredded cabbage
- 1 Cup of chopped onion
- 2 tablespoons of vegetable oil
- 1 Minced garlic clove
- 1 Package of 20 egg rolls wrappers
- 2 Tablespoons of oil

Instructions

1. Mix all your ingredients together except for the wrappers and the oil in a large bowl
2. Set your ingredients aside to marinate for about 30 minutes
3. Divide the filling between the wrappers; then fold it as directed on the package
4. Spray a baking pan with the oil and arrange the egg rolls in the dish
5. Bake the rolls for about 20 minutes in a preheated oven at a temperature of about 350° F
6. When the time is up; remove the pan from the oven
7. Serve and enjoy your eggrolls.

Nutrition Information

Calories: 159, Fats: 10g, Carbs: 7.2g, Fiber: 1.2g, Potassium: 114mg, Sodium: 152mg, Phosphorous: 56mg, Protein: 10g

Spicy beef meatballs

(Prep time: 7 Mins|Cook Time: 20 Mins| Servings: 9)

Ingredients:

- 2 Tablespoons of avocado oil
- ¼ Cup of chopped onion
- 1 Pound of lean ground chuck
- 1/3 Cup of fine dry bread crumbs
- ¼ Cup of chopped fresh parsley
- 1/8 Teaspoon of nutmeg
- ¼ Cup of liquid non-dairy creamer

- 1 Beaten egg white
- ½ Cup of finely chopped cranberries
- 2 Teaspoons of dry mustard
- 1/8 teaspoon of cayenne pepper
- ½ Cup of grape jelly
- 1 Teaspoon of lemon juice

Instructions

1. Coat a baking pan with cooking spray and place it over a medium high heat, then add in the onion and sauté your ingredients until it becomes tender
2. Combine the onion with the next 6 ingredients in a large bowl; then shape the mixture into about 35 meatballs
3. Place the meatballs over a baking sheet with the sides very well coated with cooking spray
4. Beak the meatballs for about 18 minutes at a temperature of about 375° F
5. In the meantime; prepare the sauce by mixing the cranberries with the remaining ingredients in a small pan
6. Cook your ingredients over a medium high heat for a few minutes
7. Place the meatballs in a serving dish
8. Serve and enjoy your snack!

Nutrition Information

Calories: 128, Fats: 11g, Carbs: 1g, Fiber: 0.1g, Potassium: 98mg, Sodium: 38mg, Phosphorous: 44mg, Protein 6g

Oven baked Buffalo wings

(Prep time: 5 Mins|Cook Time: 35 Mins| Servings: 8-9)

Ingredients:

- 8 tablespoons of unsalted almond butter
- ¼ Cup of roasted red pepper sauce
- 1 Tablespoon of olive oil
- ½ Teaspoon of garlic powder
- ½ Teaspoon of dried Italian seasoning blend
- 23 chicken wing drummettes

Instructions

1. Preheat your oven to a temperature of 400° F.
2. Melt the butter in a medium pan over a medium high heat
3. Add the red pepper sauce, the olive oil, the garlic powder and the Italian seasonings; then stir very well
4. Remove the saucepan from the heat and put the chicken wings in a baking pan
5. Pour the sauce over the wings and bake all together for about 30 minutes
6. Serve and enjoy your appetizer

Nutrition Information

Calories: 164, Fats: 11g, Carbs: 8g, Fiber: 1g, Potassium: 105mg, Sodium: 64mg, Phosphorous: 61mg, Protein 8g

Apple Dip

(Prep time: 4 Mins|Cook Time: 5 Mins| Servings: 2)

Ingredients:

- 8 Ounces of unsalted cream cheese
- ¾ Cup of stevia
- ½ teaspoon of vanilla extract

Instructions

1. Set the cream cheese out for about 20 minutes at the room temperature to soften it.
2. With a hand-held mixer, combine the cream cheese with the stevia and the vanilla
3. Mix your ingredients very well; then serve and enjoy your dip with apple slices

Nutrition Information

Calories: 154, Fats: 10g, Carbs: 12g, Fiber: 0.1g, Potassium: 57mg, Sodium: 107mg, Phosphorous: 31mg, Protein 4g

Frozen Cranberry salad

(Prep time: 4 Mins|Cook Time: 5 Mins| Servings: 2)

Ingredients:

- 1 Package of 8 oz of cream cheese
- ½ Pint of whipped whipping cream
- ½ teaspoon of vanilla extract
- 1 can of 16-oz of cranberry sauce

Instructions

1. Whip the cream cheese with a beater until it becomes fluffy.
2. Fold in the vanilla, the whipped cream and the cranberry sauce
3. Place the obtained mixture in a pan and freeze it for about 1 hour
4. Cut into squares; then serve and enjoy your salad!

Nutrition Information

Calories: 125, Fats: 8g, Carbs: 10g, Fiber: 0.8g, Potassium: 63mg, Sodium: 99mg, Phosphorous: 46mg, Protein 3g

Beef Meatloaf

(Prep time: 5 Mins|Cook Time: 55 Mins| Servings: 5)

Ingredients:

- 1 and ½ pounds of lean ground beef
- ¾ Cup of Panko breadcrumbs
- 2 Tablespoons of fresh oregano
- 1 and ½ tablespoons of parsley flakes
- 1 tablespoon of onion powder
- 1 teaspoon of fresh ground black pepper
- ¾ teaspoon of garlic powder
- 1 large omega-3 egg

Directions

1. Preheat your oven to a temperature of about 350 degrees F
2. In a bowl, use both your hands and mix all your ingredients together
3. Shape the mixture of the meat into the form of a loaf; then place it in a baking pan
4. Bake the meatloaf in the oven at a temperature of about 350°F for 50 to 55 minutes.
5. Slice the meatloaf; then serve and enjoy your meatloaf!

Nutrition Information

Calories: 177, Fats: 9g, Carbs: 11g, Fiber: 0.59g, Potassium: 99mg, Sodium: 55mg, Phosphorous: 68mg, Protein 13g

Chicken and grape salad

(Prep time: 5 Mins|Cook Time: 5 Mins| Servings: 3)

Ingredients:

- ¼ Cup of avocado oil
- 4 tablespoons of frozen thawed lemonade concentrate
- ¼ Teaspoon of ground ginger
- ¼ Teaspoon of curry powder
- 1/8 teaspoon of garlic powder
- 1 and ½ cups of cooked diced chicken
- 1 and ½ cups of halved grapes
- ½ Cup of sliced celery

Instructions:

1. Combine the oil with the lemonade concentrate and the spices in a large bowl
2. Add the remaining ingredients and toss it very well together
3. Let your ingredients chill for about 15 minutes
4. Serve and enjoy your salad!

Nutrition Information

Calories: 251, Fats: 15g, Carbs: 11.9g, Fiber: 1.8g, Potassium: 234mg, Sodium: 57mg, Phosphorous: 119mg, Protein 17g

Artichoke dip

(Prep time: 5 Mins|Cook Time: 20 Mins| Servings: 2)

Ingredients:

- 8 ounces of unsalted cream cheese
- 1 tablespoon of onion
- 1 teaspoon of lemon juice
- 2 teaspoons of Worcestershire sauce
- 1/8 teaspoon of black pepper
- 1/8 teaspoon of cayenne pepper
- 2 tablespoons of 1% low-fat milk
- 6 Ounces of crab meat

Instructions:

1. Preheat your oven to a temperature of 375° F; then set the cream cheese to soften and finely mince the onion
2. Put the softened cream cheese in a medium bowl.
3. Add the lemon juice with the onion, the Worcestershire sauce, the black pepper and the cayenne pepper.
4. Mix well your ingredients very well; then stir in the milk.
5. Add the crab meat and stir your ingredients very well until everything is completely blended.
6. Put the mixture in an oven-safe tray and bake while uncovered for about 15 minutes
7. Serve and enjoy your dip!

Nutrition Information

Calories: 180, Fats: 11g, Carbs: 3g, Fiber: 1.3g, Potassium: 92mg, Sodium: 191mg, Phosphorous: 68mg, Protein 17g

Oven baked okra

(Prep time: 3 Mins|Cook Time: 10 Mins| Servings: 4)

Ingredients:

- 1 pound of fresh okra
- 1 teaspoon of olive oil
- ¼ teaspoon of red pepper flakes
- ¼ Teaspoon of ground turmeric, coriander, thyme and lemon grass
- 2 Teaspoons of fresh lemon juice
- 2 tablespoons of chopped fresh parsley

Instructions:

1. Heat the oven to a temperature of 450° degrees and spray a baking sheet with cooking spray
2. Rinse the okra and pat it dry very well with clean paper towels
3. Trim both the stems and the tips of the okra; then slice it into halves in lengthwise way
4. Add the okra to a bowl and toss it with the olive oil, the red pepper flakes and the herbs; then add in the spices
5. Put the okra in a single layer over the baking sheet
6. Bake the okra for about 8 to10 minutes
7. Drizzle with the lemon juice; then garnish with the fresh parsley
8. Serve and enjoy your snack!

Nutrition Information

Calories: 90, Fats: 5g, Carbs: 7g, Fiber: 3.5g, Potassium: 169mg, Sodium: 51mg, Phosphorous: 89mg, Protein 4g

Stuffed Celery

(Prep time: 5 Mins|Cook Time: 5 Mins| Servings: 8)

Ingredients:

- 8 Washed celery stalks with then ends cut off
- 3 Tablespoons of non-fat or low-fat Greek yogurt
- 5 Tablespoons of diced red diced bell pepper
- 1 pinch of ground pepper
- 1 Tablespoon of finely chopped fresh basil
- 1 Tablespoon of finely chopped fresh chives
- 4 Omega-3 peeled eggs
- 1 Tablespoon of lemon juice

Instructions:

1. In a medium bowl, mix the yogurt with the pepper, the basil and the chives
2. Chop the eggs into fine pieces or slice it with an egg slicer
3. Add the eggs to the mixture of the yogurt
4. Add the lemon juice
5. Stuff the celery with the egg salad you have prepared; then sprinkle with the peppers and refrigerate for 10 minutes
6. Serve and enjoy your snack!

Nutrition Information

Calories: 76, Fats: 6g, Carbs: 3g, Fiber: 0.8g, Potassium: 144mg, Sodium: 69mg, Phosphorous: 37mg, Protein 2.3g

Almond cranberry stuffed celery sticks

(Prep time: 5 Mins|Cook Time: 5 Mins| Servings: 4)

Ingredients:

- 4 Medium cut celery ribs
- 4 tablespoons of mixed berry whipped cream cheese
- 24 dried cranberries
- 11 whole dry roasted and unsalted whole almonds

Instructions:

1. Start by trimming the ends of the celery ribs; then fill each of the ribs with 1 tablespoon of whipped cream cheese
2. Fill each of the celery ribs with 1 tablespoon of the whipped cream cheese.
3. Cut each of the celery ribs into 3 to 4 pieces according to the length
4. Top each of the celery rib pieces with 2 dried cranberries and 1 almond.
5. Refrigerate for about 10 minutes; then serve and enjoy your snack!

Nutrition Information

Calories: 72, Fats: 5.6g, Carbs: 3g, Fiber: 0.8g, Potassium: 138mg, Sodium: 65mg, Phosphorous: 33mg, Protein 2g

Cucumber and Onion dip

(Prep time: 3 Mins|Cook Time: 4 Mins| Servings: 4)

Ingredients:

- 8 Ounces of cream cheese
- 1 Medium cucumber
- 1 teaspoon of onion
- 1 tablespoon of lemon juice
- 1/8 teaspoon of green food colouring

Instructions:

1. Set the cream cheese out of the refrigerator to soften.
2. Peel the cucumber, seed it; then and finely mince it
3. Mix the cream cheese, the onion, the lemon juice and the green food colouring in a medium bowl and blend your ingredients until it becomes smooth.
4. Fold the cucumber into the mixture until it becomes evenly blended.

Nutrition Information

Calories: 120, Fats: 9g, Carbs: 8.5g, Fiber: 1.1g, Potassium: 138mg, Sodium: 65mg, Phosphorous: 33mg, Protein 1.3g

Oven Baked Wontons

(Prep time: 10 Mins|Cook Time: 15 Mins| Servings: 10)

Ingredients:

- 1 Ounce of lean cooked ham
- 2 tablespoons of green onions
- 2 tablespoons of sweet red pepper
- 5 large omega-3 eggs
- 1 tablespoon of all-purpose white flour
- 25 wonton wrappers

Instructions:

1. Preheat your oven to a temperature of about 350° F.
2. Finely chop the ham, the green onion and the red peppers
3. In a bowl, whisk all together the eggs, the ham, the onions, the pepper and the flour until it is very well combined and set the mixture aside
4. Lightly grease about 24 miniature muffin cups with non-stick cooking spray.
5. Line the cups wrappers with cooking spray; then spoon the mixture of the eggs into the wonton cups and divide the mixture evenly between the cups
6. Bake the wontons for about 15 minutes in your preheated oven
7. Serve and enjoy your snack!

Nutrition Information

Calories: 92, Fats: 6g, Carbs: 5.3g, Fiber: 0.9g, Potassium: 47mg, Sodium: 95mg, Phosphorous: 55mg, Protein 4g

Oven Baked Eggplant Fries

(Prep time: 5 Mins|Cook Time: 40 Mins| Servings: 3)

Ingredients:

- 1 Large eggplant
- 1 Low sodium veggie broth low sodium
- ½ teaspoon of ground black pepper
- 1 teaspoon of smoked paprika
- 2 teaspoons of stevia
- 1 Cup of almond meal
- 2 tablespoons of nutritional yeast
- 1 Tablespoon of lemon juice

Instructions:

1. Preheat your oven to a temperature of 400°F
2. Wash the eggplants and cut it into thin sicks
3. Put the eggplant pieces in a medium bowl; then sprinkle with the veggie broth, the lemon juice, the pepper, the paprika and the stevia and mix very well
4. Place the almond meal and the nutritional yeast in a separate bowl and mix your ingredients very well; then place the eggplant pieces in a bowl with almond meal; then toss very well
5. Place the eggplant pieces over a baking sheet covered with a parchment paper
6. Bake the eggplant pieces in the preheated oven for about 40 minutes
7. Serve and enjoy your oven baked eggplant pieces!

Nutrition Information

Calories: 166, Fats: 11.7g, Carbs: 6g, Fiber: 1.3g, Potassium: 104mg, Sodium: 99mg, Phosphorous: 75mg, Protein 9g

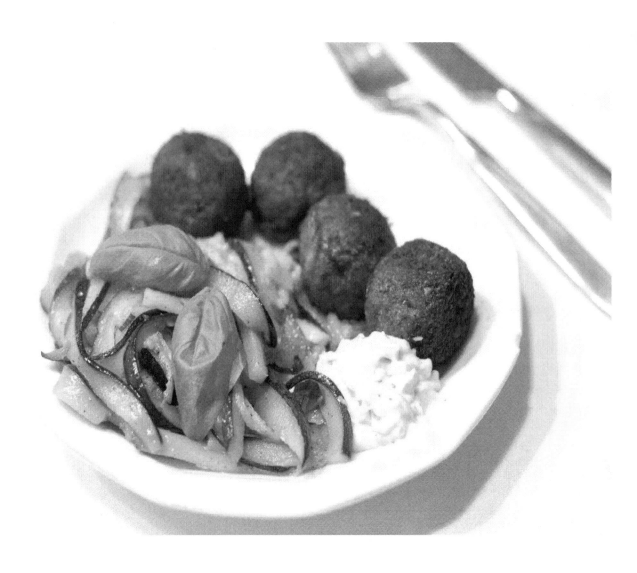

Chapter 5 Dinner Recipes

Mushroom Pizza

(Prep time: 7 Mins|Cook Time: 10 Mins| Servings: 4)

Ingredients:

- 1 Medium, flat Lavash bread
- ½ teaspoon of minced garlic
- 1 Diced, shredded onion
- 6 Diced capsicum rings
- ¼ Cup of sliced fresh mushrooms
- 1 Cup of grated mozzarella cheese
- 2 tablespoons of torn basil
- 2 teaspoons of pine nuts

Instructions:

1. Pre-heat your oven to a temperature of 360° F
2. Spray your tray with cooking spray
3. Puree the garlic with a little bit of oil and spread the mixture over the bread with the rest of the ingredients
4. Sprinkle with mozzarella cheese
5. Cook your pizza in your oven for about 10 minutes at a temperature of 360°F
6. When your pizza is perfectly cooked, slice it into quarters
7. Serve and enjoy your pizza!

Nutrition Information

Calories: 149, Fats: 10.3g, Carbs: 6.1g, Fiber: 0.9g, Potassium: 210mg, Sodium: 165mg, Phosphorous: 111mg, Protein 8g

Chicken Burgers with Sage and Apple

(Prep time: 10 Mins|Cook Time: 20 Mins| Servings: 6)

Ingredients:

- 1 Large apple
- 1 Cup of minced onion
- 2 tbsp of fresh sage
- ¼ tsp of ground allspice
- 2 Minced garlic cloves garlic
- 1 tsp of pepper
- 1 Lightly beaten omega-3 egg
- 1 Pound of ground chicken

Instructions

1. Grate the apple with the skin on and mix it with the onion, the sage, the allspice, the garlic, the pepper and the beaten egg
2. Add in the ground chicken and stir your ingredients until it become very well combined
3. Shape the meat into 1 log; then cover it with a wax paper and let it cool in the refrigerator for about 2 hours
4. Cut the log into about 8 pieces; then flatter it into pieces of ½ inch of thickness each
5. Panfry the patties in a very small quantity of oil in a non-stick skillet for about 5 minutes
6. Set the mini burgers aside to cools
7. Serve and enjoy your mini burgers!

Nutrition Information

Calories : 295, Fats: 22g, Carbs: 10.3g, Fiber: 1.5g, Potassium: 189mg, Sodium: 125mg, Phosphorous: 88g, Protein 13.8g

Turkey Spicy Fajitas

(Prep time: 15 Mins|Cook Time: 10 Mins| Servings: 10)

Ingredients:

- 1 Pound of boneless turkey breast
- ¼ teaspoon of ground black pepper
- 1 Minced garlic clove
- 1 teaspoon of Chilli powder
- 2 tablespoons of lime juice
- 1 tablespoon of chopped fresh cilantro
- 1 tablespoon of oil
- 2 tablespoons of chopped fresh cilantro
- 1 tablespoon of chopped red onion
- ¼ teaspoon of minced garlic
- 10 flour tortillas of 7 inch each
- 3 Cups of shredded lettuce
- 1 Cup of chopped red bell pepper

Instructions

1. Sprinkle the turkey with the ground pepper, 1 minced garlic clove, the chilli powder, the lime juice, 1 tablespoon of cilantro and the oil. Turn the turkey to coat it very well
2. Cover the turkey with a lid or a plastic wrap and set it aside to marinate for about 2 and ½ hours
3. Combine the red pepper with the cilantro, the onion and about ¼ teaspoon of garlic in a bowl; then let the mixture stand for about 1 hour
4. Broil the turkey for about 10 minutes from the heat per each side; then cut it into strips
5. Wrap the tortillas into an aluminium foil and let it warm in the oven for about 8 minutes
6. Serve and enjoy your dinner with the prepared onion and pepper mixture!

Nutrition Information

Calories: 321, Fats: 24g, Carbs: 12.2g, Fiber: 2.6g, Potassium: 204mg, Sodium: 192mg, Phosphorous: 129g, Protein 14g

Pork Souvlaki

(Prep time: 5 Mins|Cook Time: 20 Mins| Servings: 3)

Ingredients:

- 1 Pound of pork; cut into cubes
- ¼ Cup of olive oil
- 3 tbsp of lemon juice
- 1 tsp of ground oregano
- ¼ tsp of black pepper
- 1 Large, minced garlic clove

Instructions

1. Trim any fat from the pork and cut it into cubes; then set it aside
2. Add the remaining ingredients to a bowl and mix very well
3. Add the pork to the marinade mixture in the bowl and coat the pork very well with it; then set it aside for about 2 to 3 hours
4. Stir fry the pork meat in a large pan over a medium high heat for about 7 to 10 minutes
5. Place the pork meat on skewers and grill it over a medium high heat for about 8 to 10 minutes; and make sure to turn once during the grilling
6. Serve and enjoy your dinner!

Nutrition Information

Calories: 274, Fats: 18g, Carbs: 7g, Fiber: 1.12g, Potassium: 197mg, Sodium:156mg, Phosphorous: 129g, Protein 21g

Steamed Talipa Dish with Lemon Juice

(Prep time: 10 Mins|Cook Time: 20 Mins| Servings: 4-5)

Ingredients:

- 4 to 5 tilapia fillets
- 3 tablespoons of fresh lemon juice
- 1 tablespoon of olive oil
- 1 Finely chopped garlic clove
- 1 Teaspoon of dried parsley flakes pepper

Instructions

1. Preheat your oven to a temperature of about oven to about 375°F
2. Spray a baking pan with non-stick cooking spray and set it aside
3. Rinse the tilapia fillets under the cool water, and pat it dry with clean paper towels.
4. Place the fillets in the baking dish; then pour the lemon juice over the fillets and drizzle with oil on top
5. Sprinkle with the garlic, the parsley, and the pepper.
6. Bake the Talipa in your preheated oven for about 30 minutes
7. Serve and enjoy your dinner!

Nutrition Information

Calories: 227, Fats: 15.8g, Carbs: 8g, Fiber: 1.4g, Potassium: 242mg, Sodium: 59mg, Phosphorous: 95g, Protein 13g

Salmon with Horseradish

(Prep time: 7 Mins|Cook Time: 18 Mins| Servings: 3)

Ingredients:

- 4 Pieces of 6 Oz of skinless salmon fillet
- 1 Tablespoon of lemon juice
- 1 pinch of ground black pepper
- ¼ Cup of fresh white bread crumbs
- 1 tablespoon of prepared horseradish
- 1 tablespoon of chopped fresh flat-leaf parsley
- 2 tablespoons of olive oil
- 4 cups of mixed greens
- 2 teaspoons of white wine vinegar

Instructions

1. Heat your oven to a temperature of about 400º F.
2. Season the salmon with about ½ tablespoon of lemon juice and about ¼ teaspoon of pepper; then place your ingredients together over a baking sheet
3. In a medium bowl, combine the horseradish, the bread crumbs, the parsley, and about 1 tablespoon of the olive oil.
4. Spread the mixture over the salmon and roast it for about 13 to 15 minutes
5. In a medium bowl, combine the vinegar with the greens, the remaining tablespoon of olive oil, and the remaining lemon juice
6. Serve with the baked salmon
7. Enjoy your dinner!

Nutrition Information

Calories: 282, Fats: 19g, Carbs: 5.6g, Fiber: 0.9g, Potassium: 263mg, Sodium:89mg, Phosphorous: 85g, Protein 22g

Renal Diet Pilaf

(Prep time: 5 Mins|Cook Time: 15 Mins| Servings: 2-3)

Ingredients:

- 1 Cup of uncooked basmati rice
- 2 Tablespoons of dried unsweetened cranberries
- 1 to 2 bay leaves
- 1 Small cinnamon stick
- ½ Teaspoon of black cumin
- 2 Tablespoons of olive oil
- 2 Cups of water

Instructions

1. Soak the rice and all the ingredients for about 40 to 45 minutes at the room temperature.
2. Place the ingredients into a microwave for about 12 minutes at its full power
3. Let the rice cool for 5 minutes for about 5 minutes
4. Serve and enjoy your dinner!

Nutrition Information

Calories: 190, Fats: 16g, Carbs: 8.2g, Fiber: 2.7g, Potassium: 71mg, Sodium: 34mg, Phosphorous: 74g, Protein 3g

Lamb Runza

(Prep time: 10 Mins|Cook Time: 30 Mins| Servings: 6)

Ingredients:

- 1 Pound of ground lamb
- ¼Cup of onion
- 1/8 tsp of black pepper
- 4 Cups of shredded cabbage
- 1 Frozen loaf of bread dough
- 1 teaspoon of vinegar

Instructions

1. Start nu thaw ing the frozen bread dough; then preheat your oven to a temperature of about 350° F
2. Boil the shredded cabbage in hot water
3. Cook the onion, the ground lamb and the pepper for about 5 minutes
4. Add the boiled cabbage to the mixture of the burger.
5. Roll the dough of bread in a rectangular shape; then cut into the shape you want
6. Place the burger mixture over the bread into a rectangular; then fold over and pinch the edges
7. Bake the bread for about 25 minutes
8. Serve and enjoy your dinner hot!

Nutrition Information

Calories: 255, Fats: 19g, Carbs: 10.1g, Fiber: 2.33g, Potassium: 195mg, Sodium:98mg, Phosphorous: 114g, Protein 10.5g

Onion Pie

(Prep time: 10 Mins|Cook Time: 40 Mins| Servings: 7)

Ingredients:

- 1 and ½ cups of crushed Ritz crackers
- 1/3 Cup of avocado oil
- 2 Teaspoons of olive oil
- 2 Cups of sliced sweet onions,
- 1 Teaspoon of lemon juice
- 1/8 tsp of black pepper
- 2 Large omega-3 eggs
- ¼ Cup of mozzarella cheese
- ¾ Cup of half and half

Instructions

1. Preheat your oven to a temperature of 350°F.
2. Mix the Ritz crackers and about 1/3 cup of avocado oil
3. Press the mixture in a pie pan of about 9 inch
4. Heat a skillet over a medium high heat; then add the olive oil to it and sauté the onions for about 2 minutes
5. Cook the onions until it becomes clear; then spread it into the crust.
6. Crack the eggs in a bowl and combine it with the half and half
7. Add the pepper
8. Pour the mixture over the onions then spread the cheese over the top
9. Bake for about 30 minutes or until set.

Nutrition Information

Calories: 175, Fats: 13g, Carbs: 8g, Fiber: 1.5g, Potassium: 119mg, Sodium: 36mg, Phosphorous: 105g, Protein 6.3g

Pepper Pizza

(Prep time: 15 Mins|Cook Time: 25 Mins| Servings: 5)

Ingredients:

INGREDIENTS FOR THE PIZZA:

- 1 Pita, Greek style
- 2 tbsp of roasted red pepper sauce
- ¼ Cup of cooked ground beef
- 1 tbsp of diced green pepper
- 1 tbsp of diced onion, diced
- 2 tbsp of diced brie
- 2 tbsp of grated mozzarella

INGREDIENTS TO PREPARE THE PEPPER SAUCE:

- 1 roasted whole red pepper
- 2 Garlic cloves
- 1 Pinch of ground black pepper
- 1 tsp of olive oil

Instructions

1. Preheat your oven to a temperature of 350°F; then place the pita over a baking sheet and prepare the pepper sauce and to do that roast the pepper in a broiler or barbecue it until it the skin becomes black
2. Let the pepper cool; then peel it and puree the peppers with the garlic, the black pepper and the olive oil in a food processor
3. Spread the sauce over the pita; then add pepper slices and top with the green pepper, the beef, the onion and the cheeses and bake for about 10 minutes
4. Slice your pizza; then serve and enjoy it hot

Nutrition Information

Calories: 170.3, Fats: 9g, Carbs: 11g, Fiber: 2.4g, Potassium: 81mg, Sodium: 67mg, Phosphorous: 91g, Protein 11g

Baked Dilly Pickerel

(Prep time: 5 Mins|Cook Time: 15 Mins| Servings: 3)

Ingredients:

- 4 Fillets of pickerel, about 4 oz

For the dilly Sauce

- ½ package of whipped cream cheese
- 4 Minced garlic cloves
- ½ Diced small onion
- 3 tbsp of fresh or dried dill
- ½ tsp of ground pepper

Instructions

1. Preheat your oven to a temperature of 350°F.
2. Mix the ingredients of the dilly sauce very well to make a paste.
3. Line a baking pan with a tin foil; then set the fish and spread the dilly sauce on its top
4. Cover the fish with an aluminium foil tin and bake it for about 15 minutes in the oven
5. Serve and enjoy your dinner!

Nutrition Information

Calories: 295.6, Fats: 18.7g, Carbs: 11g, Fiber: 2.2g, Potassium: 140mg, Sodium: 6.8mg, Phosphorous: 58g, Protein 20.7g

Rice Salad

(Prep time: 10 Mins|Cook Time: 20 Mins| Servings: 2)
Ingredients:

- 1 Cup of olive oil
- ½ Cup of balsamic vinegar
- 1 teaspoon of lemon juice
- ¾ teaspoons of black pepper
- 3 Minced garlic cloves
- ½ teaspoon of dried basil
- ½ teaspoon of dried oregano
- ½ Cup of fresh parsley
- 2 cups of bell peppers

- ½ Cup of chopped red onion
- 1 Cup of frozen artichoke hearts
- 1/3 Cup of fresh dill weed
- 6 Cups of cooked white rice
- 1 Pound of cooked shrimp
- ½ Cup of dried cranberries
- 8 Ounces of canned pineapple chunks
- 1 Cup of frozen green peas

Instructions

1. To make the dressing, whisk all together the oil with the vinegar, the salt, the pepper, the minced garlic, the basil, the oregano and about ¼ cup of chopped parsley; then set the mixture aside.
2. Chop the red bell peppers and the onion; then mince the dill weed
3. Cook your ingredients and quarter the artichoke hearts.
4. In a large bowl combine the rice with the shrimp, the bell peppers, the onion, the artichoke hearts, and ½ cup of minced parsley, the dill, the cranberries, the pineapple and the green peas.
5. Stir the dressing into the salad and let it chill for about 2 hours to marinate.
6. Serve and enjoy your dinner over a bed of lettuce!

Nutrition Information

Calories: 165.4, Fats: 11g, Carbs: 8g, Fiber: 0.89g, Potassium: 181mg, Sodium:99mg, Phosphorous: 75g, Protein 8g

Baked Eggplant Tray

(Prep time: 10 Mins|Cook Time: 20 Mins| Servings: 2)

Ingredients:

- 3 Cups of eggplant
- 3 large omega-3 eggs
- ½ Cup of liquid non-dairy creamer
- 1 teaspoon of vinegar
- 1 Teaspoon of lemon juice
- ½ teaspoon of pepper
- ¼ teaspoon of sage
- ½ Cup of white breadcrumbs
- 1 tablespoon of margarine

Instructions

1. Preheat your oven to a temperature of about 350° F
2. Peel the eggplant and cut it into pieces
3. Place the eggplant pieces in a large pan; then cover it with water and let boil until it becomes tender
4. Drain the eggplants and mash it very well
5. Combine the beaten eggs with the non-dairy creamer, the vinegar, the lemon juice, the pepper and the sage with the mashed eggplant; then place it into a greased baking tray
6. Mix the melted margarine with the breadcrumbs.
7. Top you tray with the breadcrumbs and bake it for about 20 minutes
8. Set the tray aside to cool for about 5 minutes
9. Serve and enjoy your dinner!

Nutrition Information

Calories: 126, Fats: 8g, Carbs: 4.7g, Fiber: 1.6g, Potassium: 224mg, Sodium: 143mg, Phosphorous: 115g, Protein 7.3g

Cranberry Chutney

(Prep time: 5 Mins|Cook Time: 25 Mins| Servings: 3)

Ingredients:

- 1/3 Cup of finely chopped shallot
- 1 tablespoon of unsalted almond butter
- 6 oz of fresh cranberries, about 2 cups
- ½ Cup of stevia
- 1/3 Cup of water
- 1 tablespoon of cider vinegar
- ¾ Teaspoon of cracked black pepper
- ¼ teaspoon of lemon juice

Instructions

1. Cook the shallot in the almond butter in a heavy pan over a medium heat and stir from time to time for about 5 minutes
2. Stir in the remaining ingredients and let simmer while stirring from time to time; but this time the pan should be uncovered for about 20 minutes
3. Let the chutney cool for about 5 minutes
4. Serve and enjoy your dish!

Nutrition Information

Calories: 128.4, Fats: 8.3g, Carbs: 6.9g, Fiber: 1.9g, Potassium: 118mg, Sodium: 184mg, Phosphorous: 65g, Protein 6g

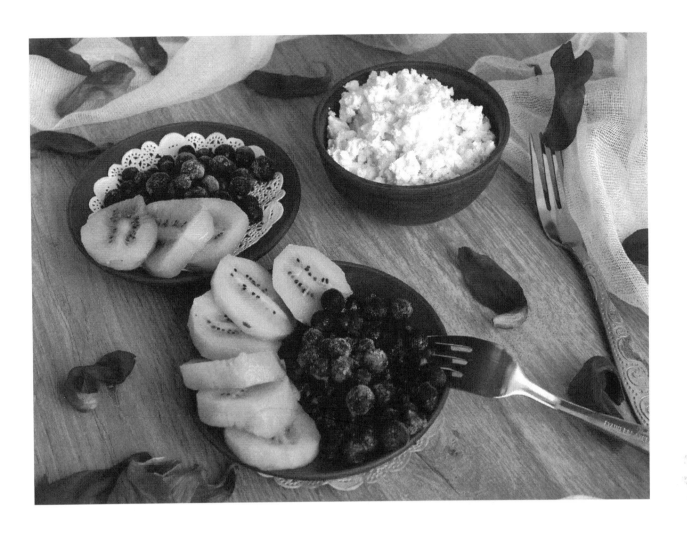

Chapter 6 Dessert Recipes

Apple Cookies

(Prep time: 15 Mins|Cook Time: 12 Mins| Servings: 12)

Ingredients:

- ½ Cup of shortening
- 1/2 Cup of almond butter
- ½ Cup of stevia
- ½ Cup of brown sugar
- 1 Omega-3 egg
- ½ tsp of vanilla Extract
- 1 and ½ cups of All-Purpose Flour
- ½ Tsp of baking Soda
- 1/2 tsp of salt
- 1/2 tsp of ground Cinnamon
- 1 Cup of peeled and grated apple

Instructions

1. Cream the shortening in a bowl together with the butter and the stevia and the brown sugar
2. When your mixture becomes fluffy, beat in the egg and the vanilla; then combine your dry ingredients
3. Gradually pour the creamed mixture into the dry ingredients and mix very well
4. Stir in the apple; then drop rounded spoonfuls of about 2 inches over a greased baking sheet
5. Bake your cookies over a the baking sheet for about 12 minutes
6. Let your cookies cool for about 10 minutes
7. Serve and enjoy your cookies!

Nutrition Information

Calories: 85, Fats: 4.8g, Carbs: 6g, Fiber: 1.1g, Potassium: 96mg, Sodium: 129mg, Phosphorous: 47g, Protein 4.1g

Raspberry Muffins

(Prep time: 10 Mins|Cook Time: 20 Mins| Servings: 10)

Ingredients:

- 1 and 1/3 cups of flour
- 1 and ½ teaspoons of baking soda
- 1 Cup of fresh or frozen raspberries
- ¼ Cup of margarine
- ½ Cup of stevia
- 1 Omega-3 egg
- ½ cup of liquid non-dairy creamer
- ¼ Cup of stevia
- ¼ Cup of flour
- 2 tablespoons of margarine
- 2 teaspoons of cinnamon

Instructions

1. Preheat your oven to a temperature of 375°F.
2. Line a 16 muffin cups with paper liners; then combine about 1 and 1/3 cups of flour with the baking soda in a small bowl and stir in the raspberries
3. In a separate medium bowl; beat the ¼ cup of margarine with the brown sugar and the egg and blender very well
4. Add in the flour and stir until your mixture becomes smooth
5. Spoon the batter in about 16 muffin cups
6. In another bowl, mix the stevia with ¼ cup of flour, 2 tablespoons of margarine and the cinnamon; then sprinkle it over the muffins
7. Bake your muffins for about 15 to 18 minutes
8. Serve and enjoy your muffins!

Nutrition Information

Calories: 156.2, Fats: 10g, Carbs: 13g, Fiber: 0.8g, Potassium: 56mg, Sodium: 111mg, Phosphorous: 69g, Protein 3g

Kidney-friendly Unsalted Pretzels

(Prep time: 15 Mins|Cook Time: 15 Mins| Servings: 12)

Ingredients:

- 1 Package of dry yeast
- ¾ Cup of warm water
- 1 Tablespoon of stevia
- 2 Cups of flour
- 2 tablespoons of almond milk
- 1 tablespoon of sesame seeds

Instructions

1. Mix the dry yeast with warm water; then add in the stevia and beat in the flour
2. Knead your dough until it becomes smooth for about 10 minutes
3. Place the dough over a floured surface and divide it into about 12 pieces
4. Roll the pieces into ropes of about 12 inches each
5. Shape each dough rope into the form of a pretzel; then place it over a greased baking sheet and brush it with milk
6. Sprinkle the sesame seeds; then bake your pretzels at a temperature of about 425° F for about 12 to 15 minutes
7. Let the pretzels cool for about 5 minutes
8. Serve and enjoy!

Nutrition Information

Calories: 142, Fats: 8g Carbs: 13g, Fiber: 1, Potassium: 61mg, Sodium: 3mg, Phosphorous: 48g, Protein 3.5g

Vanilla Custard

(Prep time: 5 Mins|Cook Time: 30 Mins| Servings: 3)

Ingredients:

- ½ Cup of low fat (2%) milk
- 1 Large vegan egg
- 1/8 teaspoon of nutmeg
- 1/8 teaspoon of vanilla
- 2 Tablespoons of stevia
- Artificial sweetener

Instructions

1. Scald the milk then let it cool slightly.
2. Break the egg into a small bowl and beat it with the nutmeg
3. Add the scalded milk, the vanilla and the sweetener to taste; then mix very well
4. Place the bowl in a baking pan filled with ½ deep of water and bake for about 30 minutes at a temperature of about 325° F
5. Serve and enjoy your custard!

Nutrition Information

Calories: 167.3, Fats: 9g, Carbs: 11g, Fiber: 1.8g, Potassium: 249mg, Sodium: 124mg, Phosphorous: 205g, Protein 10g

Almond Cookies

(Prep time: 7 Mins|Cook Time: 10 Mins| Servings: 10)

Ingredients:

- 1 Cup of softened margarine
- 1 Cup of stevia
- 1 Vegan egg
- 3 Cups of white flour
- 1 teaspoon of baking soda
- 1 teaspoon of almond extract

Instructions

1. Cream the margarine in a bowl; then add the stevia to it and beat very well
2. Sift your dry ingredients and add it to the creamed mixture
3. Add in the almond extract and mix very well.
4. Roll the dough into balls of about ¾ inches in diameter.
5. Make a small hole in each of the cookies and bake for about 12 minutes at a temperature of 400° F
6. Let the cookies cool for about 10 minutes
7. Serve and enjoy your dessert!

Nutrition Information

Calories: 88, Fats: 5g, Carbs: 8g, Fiber: 0.8g, Potassium: 28mg, Sodium: 99mg, Phosphorous: 30g, Protein 2.3g

Chocolate Chip Cookies

(Prep time: 7 Mins|Cook Time: 10 Mins| Servings: 10)

Ingredients:

- 1 Cup of flour
- ½ teaspoon of baking soda
- 1/4 Teaspoon of salt
- ½ Cup of margarine
- 4 Teaspoons of stevia
- ½ teaspoon of vanilla
- 1 Beaten vegan egg
- ½ Cup of semi-sweet chocolate chips

Instructions

1. Sift your dry ingredients all together
2. Cream the margarine; the stevia, the vanilla and the egg and whisk very well
3. Add flour mixture and beat again
4. Stir in the chocolate chips; then drop teaspoonfuls of the mixture over a greased baking sheet
5. Bake your cookies for about 10 minutes at a temperature of 375° F
6. Let your cookies cool for 5 minutes
7. Serve and enjoy your chocolate chip cookies!

Nutrition Information

Calories: 106.2, Fats: 7g, Carbs: 8.9g, Fiber: 0.3g, Potassium: 28mg, Sodium: 98mg, Phosphorous: 19g, Protein 1.5g

Fruit Compote

(Prep time: 5 Mins|Cook Time: 30 Mins| Servings: 3)

Ingredients:

- 28 oz of pear slices
- 28 oz of peach slices
- 28 oz of Pineapple chunks,

To make the cherry pie filling:

- 2 Cups of crushed almond flakes
- ¼ cup of melted margarine

Instructions

1. Wash and drain your fruits very well; then grease a baking pan with cooking spray
2. Cut your fruits into slices; then arrange the fruit slices in the bottom of your baking pan
3. Crush the Grease a 9 x 13-inch pan and layer fruit, ending with pie filling.
4. Crush the almond flakes; then mix it with the margarine and sprinkle it over the fruits
5. Bake your pie for about 30 minutes at a temperature of 350°F
6. Serve and enjoy your dessert!

Nutrition Information

Calories: 135.2, Fats: 10g, Carbs: 8.5g, Fiber: 1.3g, Potassium: 286mg, Sodium: 115mg, Phosphorous: 32g, Protein 2.5g

Puffed Cereal Bars

(Prep time: 5 Mins|Cook Time: 10 Mins| Servings: 10)

Ingredients:

- 1/3 Cup of margarine
- 1 and ½ cups of stevia
- 1 teaspoon of maple extract
- 8 Cups of puffed rice cereal

Instructions

1. In a large saucepan and over a medium high heat, melt the margarine; then stir in the stevia, the maple extract and let boil for about 7 to 10 minutes
2. Stir in the puffed rice cereal; then let the mixture cool for about 5 minutes
3. Press the mixture into a greased baking pan and let chill for about 15 minutes
4. Cut into about 20 bars
5. Serve and enjoy your dessert!

Nutrition Information

Calories: 111, Fats: 7.9g, Carbs: 6.4g, Fiber: 1.2g, Potassium: 10mg, Sodium: 26mg, Phosphorous: 15g, Protein 3g

Strawberry Ice-cream

(Prep time: 5 Mins|Cook Time: 5 Mins| Servings: 3)

Ingredients:

- 1 Package of 10-oz of unsweetened strawberries
- 1 tablespoon of lemon juice
- 1 Cup of crushed ice
- ¾ Cup of non-dairy coffee creamer
- ½ Cup of stevia

Instructions

1. Thaw the strawberries until it starts breaking up into chunks
2. Blend your ingredients until it becomes smooth
3. Pour your mixture into a dish
4. Freeze the ice cream in the dish for about 1 hour
5. Serve and enjoy your dessert!

Nutrition Information

Calories: 94.4, Fats: 6g, Carbs: 8.3g., Fiber: 0.3g, Potassium: 108mg, Sodium: 25mg, Phosphorous: 25g, Protein 1.3g

Peach Cobbler

(Prep time: 6 Mins|Cook Time: 20 Mins| Servings: 4)

Ingredients:

- ½ Cup of plain flour
- ½ Cup of stevia
- ½ Cup of coffee creamer
- 1 teaspoon of baking soda
- 2 Cups of sliced peaches

Instructions

1. Mix all together the plain flour, the stevia and the baking soda
2. Add the coffee creamer and mix very well
3. Add the peaches with its juice and mix again.
4. Pour the mixture in a baking pan
5. Bake for about 15 to 20 minutes at a temperature of about 350° F
6. Serve and enjoy your peach cobbler!

Nutrition Information

Calories: 103, Fats: 6.5g, Carbs: 8.7g, Fiber: 1g, Potassium: 156mg, Sodium: 97mg, Phosphorous: 52g, Protein 2g

Zucchini Cake

(Prep time: 10 Mins|Cook Time: 60 Mins| Servings: 5)

Ingredients:

- 4 Omega-3 eggs
- 1 Cup of avocado oil
- ½ Cup of stevia
- 2 Tablespoons of molasses
- 3 Cups of grated raw zucchini
- 3 Cups of white flour
- 1 Teaspoon of baking soda
- 1 Teaspoon of cinnamon
- ¼ Cup of chopped nuts

Instructions

1. Start by beating the eggs; then add in the oil, the stevia and the molasses
2. Add in the zucchini and blend the mixture until it is very well combined
3. Combine the flour, the baking soda and the cinnamon; then add it to your mixture
4. Blend in the nuts and bake in a greased baking pan in your oven for about 1 hour at a temperature of about 350° F
5. Slice your cake; then serve and enjoy it

Nutrition Information

Calories: 153, Fats: 11g, Carbs: 8g, Fiber: 1.23g, Potassium: 102mg, Sodium: 68mg, Phosphorous: 47g, Protein 4g

Apple Cake

(Prep time: 8 Mins|Cook Time: 60 Mins| Servings: 6)

Ingredients:

- ½ Cup of melted almond butter
- 2 Cups of stevia
- 2 large vegan eggs
- 1 tsp of vanilla extract
- 2 cups of sifted all purpose flour
- 2 Teaspoons of ground cinnamon
- 1 Teaspoon of baking soda
- 4 Large peeled and thinly sliced granny smith apples

Instructions:

1. Preheat your oven to a temperature of about 350°F.
2. Stir all together the almond butter, the stevia, the eggs and the vanilla and combine very well
3. Combine the flour with the cinnamon and the baking soda and combine very well
4. Add in the apples and spread your batter in a greased baking pan
5. Bake your batter for about 60 minutes at a temperature of 325° F
6. Slice your cake; then serve and enjoy it!

Nutrition Information

Calories: 172.4, Fats: 13g, Carbs: 8g, Fiber: 1.5g, Potassium: 126mg, Sodium: 120mg, Phosphorous: 46g, Protein 4.3g

Vanilla Low Potassium Cocoa Cake

(Prep time: 5 Mins|Cook Time: 45 Mins| Servings: 5)

Ingredients:

- 1 Cup of stevia
- 3 tbsp of cocoa
- 1 and ½ cups of white flour
- 1 tsp of baking soda
- 1 tbsp of vinegar
- 1 Teaspoon of vanilla
- ¼ Cup of coconut oil
- 1 Cup of warm water

Instructions:

1. Sift your dry ingredients into a large bowl.
2. Pour the vinegar, the vanilla, the oil and the warm water over your dry ingredients and mix very well
3. Pour your batter in a greased baking pan of about 8x8.
4. Slice your cake with a knife and make holes in it
5. Bake for about 45 minutes at a temperature of about 300° F
6. Slice your cake; serve and enjoy its succulent taste!

Nutrition Information

Calories: 156, Fats: 12g, Carbs: 6g, Fiber: 1g, Potassium: 115mg, Sodium: 130mg, Phosphorous: 56g, Protein 3g

Blueberry Cones

(Prep time: 5 Mins|Cook Time: 5 Mins| Servings: 6)

Ingredients:

- 4 Ounces of low phosphorus cream cheese
- 1 and ½ cups of whipped topping
- 1 and ¼ cups of frozen or fresh blueberries
- ¼ Cup of blueberry jam
- 6 Ice cream cones

Instructions:

1. Soften the cream cheese and place it into a bowl; then beat it with a mixer on a high speed until it becomes fluffy and smooth
2. Fold the fruits and the jam and the whipped topping into the cream cheese
3. Fill the cones and let it chill for about 2 hours
4. Serve and enjoy your dessert!

Nutrition Information

Calories: 112, Fats: 6g, Carbs: 8g, Fiber: 1.4g, Potassium: 81mg, Sodium: 95mg, Phosphorous: 40g, Protein 3.6g

Chapter 7 The 14 Day Meal Plan

Meal / Day	Breakfast	Appetizer Snack Salad	Lunch	Dessert	Dinner
Day 1	Eggs in hole	Spicy beef meatballs	Pork chops with apple	Raspberry Muffins	Chicken Burgers with Sage and Apple
Day 2	Kidney-friendly French toast	Egg Rolls	Lamb with fruit sauce	Apple Cookies	Turkey Spicy Fajitas
Day 3	Fruit and rolled oat Pancakes	Oven baked Buffalo wings	Slow Cooked chuck roast with onion	Kidney-friendly Unsalted Pretzels	Mushroom Pizza
Day 4	Deviled eggs	Apple Dip	Oven Baked Halibut	Vanilla Custard	Pork Souvlaki
Day 5	Omelet with onion and apple	Frozen Cranberry salad	Garlic Shrimp	Almond Cookies	Steamed Talipa Dish with Lemon Juice
Day 6	Breakfast Pork casserole	Chicken and grape salad	Spicy fish with peppers	Chocolate Chip Cookies	Salmon with Horseradish
Day 7	Pepper Quiche	Artichoke dip	Spicy Chicken Marsala	Fruit Compote	Renal Diet Pilaf

Meal / Day	Breakfast	Appetizer Snack Salad	Lunch	Dessert	Dinner
Day 8	Egg Benedict	Oven baked okra	Chicken Curry	Puffed Cereal Bars	Lamb Runza
Day 9	Waffles with cocoa powder	Stuffed Celery	Steak with onion	Strawberry Ice-cream	Onion Pie
Day 10	Cauliflower and broccoli gratin	Almond cranberry stuffed celery sticks	Shrimp scampi	Peach Cobbler	Pepper Pizza
Day 11	Wheat Berry bowl	Cucumber and Onion dip	Chicken Paella	Zucchini Cake	Baked Dilly Pickerel
Day 12	Unsalted, Breakfast tortillas	Oven Baked Wontons	Beef Kabobs with pepper	Apple Cake	Rice Salad
Day 13	Breakfast Couscous	Oven Baked Eggplant Fries	Pork Tenderloin with cumin	Vanilla Low Potassium Cocoa Cake	Baked Eggplant Tray
Day 14	Breakfast Berry bowl	Frozen Cranberry salad	Slow cooked chicken with lemon and oregano	Blueberry Cones	Cranberry Chutney

Conclusion

Our kidneys make an essential organ that is responsible for filtering our blood on a daily basis. However, when our kidneys start mal functioning, different organs can get affected and our body becomes unable to get rid of the excess of fluids and the toxic wastes of our body. Therefore keeping our kidneys healthy is the cornerstone of our well being, long and healthy life.

Thus when living with a chronic kidney disease, controlling what you eat and what you drink makes an important step that can help prevent your health condition from deteriorating. And this is where this book stems from. In fact, this "Cope with your kidney disease and say good bye to dialysis" has proven its efficiency in controlling all types of kidney diseases that can endanger your life and that can change your basic lifestyle forever.

This book offers 70 easy to make, delicious and succulent low phosphorus, low sodium and low potassium recipes that will help reduce any strain on your kidneys and will help you achieve better results.

And to make this book easier to read for you, I have made sure to categorize the recipes under certain subcategories like breakfast recipes, lunches, dinners, snacks, appetizers, salads and desserts. Each of the recipes you will come across offers you a wide range of 14 delicious renal diet recipes that you can see in the meal plan I have made specifically for you.

The 14 day meal plan I have included in this book will help you decide what you eat everyday without thinking too much about what you should and what you should not eat and with each recipe, you will find the recipe's nutritional information with specific Calories, protein, potassium, sodium and phosphorus. It is also recommended that you consult a renal dietician. And remember that as a kidney disease keeps progressing throughout time, your diet needs to be adjusted to the new condition. Try this book, you never know; it can save your life.

Made in the USA
Lexington, KY
13 April 2019